From the author of the best selling Tool Ki

THE NEW GP CONTRACT

How to make the most of it

Roy Lilley

Foreword by
John Chisholm

Radcliffe Medical Press

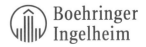
Boehringer
Ingelheim

Provided as a service to medicine by Boehringer Ingelheim

Radcliffe Medical Press Ltd
18 Marcham Road
Abingdon
Oxon OX14 1AA
United Kingdom

www.radcliffe-oxford.com
The Radcliffe Medical Press electronic catalogue and online ordering facility.
Direct sales to anywhere in the world.

British Library Cataloguing in Publication Data

A catalogue record for this book is available from the British Library.

ISBN 1 85775 879 X

Typeset by Joshua Associates Ltd, Oxford
Printed and bound by TJ International Ltd, Padstow, Cornwall

CONTENTS

FOREWORD BY JOHN CHISHOLM

Roy Lilley and I have been on the opposite sides of many debates about the NHS. So why am I writing this foreword? The answer is that both Roy and I want to see accessible guidance getting into the hands of GPs and practice teams, so that the new GP contract works.

The overwhelmingly supportive vote in June 2003 in favour of the implementation of the contract means practices and Primary Care Organisations are now urgently planning for the contract's full implementation in April next year. GPs, practices and PCOs need as much guidance as they can get – from the General Practitioners Committee, the NHS Confederation and also from books such as this. The more advice they can turn to and the earlier they can get the help they need the better. So I welcome Roy's book as a valuable – if characteristically trenchant – contribution to that advice, written in his own inimitable, cynical, sometimes knockabout and irreverent style. The book is intended for reference but also to help in brainstorming solutions and new ways of working.

Of course, and hardly surprisingly, I do not agree with Roy's every word. But I do endorse his dedication, in which he recognises that NHS professionals will bust a gut to make the new contract a success for patients. The contract would not have been worth negotiating if it did not improve services for patients – above all through the better health outcomes, the reductions in premature deaths and the improved quality of care that will result from the evidence-based quality and outcomes framework. And, unlike Roy, I do not believe it will spell the demise of the family doctor. What he wants to preserve – what he describes in this book's epilogue – I want too.

Roy is not a fan of the new contract. I am. I'm proud to have negotiated it, I'm delighted by the step change in resources for primary care, and I believe that the contract will lead to a regeneration of general practice and long overdue improvements in recruitment, retention and morale.

But despite Roy's conclusions about the contract's merits, his book is primarily an informative summary of the contract documents and a practical tool kit for putting the contract into action. I too want to see practice teams making the contract work, and this book will help many of them to do so.

John Chisholm
Chairman
General Practitioners Committee
British Medical Association
September 2003

ABOUT THE AUTHOR

Roy Lilley was formerly a visiting fellow at the Management School, Imperial College London. He is a writer and broadcaster on health and social issues and has published over two dozen books on health and health service management and related topics.

As a former NHS Trust chairman his Trust became the first to achieve BS 5750 (ISO 9001) quality accreditation for the whole of their services along with *Investors in People* approval for the whole of their HR and training strategies. The Trust agreed the only 'no-strike' deal in the NHS.

All staff took part in performance management and everyone had a personal development plan.

Roy Lilley now writes, broadcasts and works across the NHS to help with the challenges of modern management and is an enthusiast for radical policies that address the real needs of patients, professionals and the communities they serve.

Acknowledgements

I am indebted to the new contract negotiating teams who, despite the sometimes tricky and confidential nature of their work, did their utmost to keep as much as possible of what was going on in the public domain. Without that, authors like me and books like this can never be conceived of.

I am a particular admirer of the BMA website, which is stuffed full of really useful new contract information and implementation help.

Their material is the major source for this book.

DEDICATION

For ATR, who has provided excellent personal services and has never appeared to want to renegotiate the contract!

And to the army of NHS professionals who will bust a gut to make the new contract a success for patients.

GETTING THE BEST FROM THIS BOOK

Beware! This is a book with attitude. You may not agree, it might annoy you, but at least it'll get you talking! The new contract is complex and will have an impact on pretty well everyone working in primary care. The contract may be about the 'pay and rations' for GPs, but implementation is not just for GPs or practice bosses. It will take a team effort. There are big changes and big responsibilities to take on.

Use the book as a reference tool, as a help for brainstorming solutions and ideas, and for translating some of the more arcane sections into English. Look to it for commentary and opinion.

The book is aimed at helping to make the contract 'do-able'. There are:

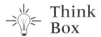 **Think Box**

Think boxes – they are there to get 'the juices flowing' and to get you thinking 'outside the box', to look at the issues from a different dimension. Some are deliberately provocative, some just for fun.

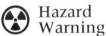 Hazard Warning

Hazard warnings, to let you know 'this bit is tricky' or could be a problem.

✓ There are **Tips**, for short cuts and bright ideas.

. . . and the inevitable ☕, a good place to sit down, make a cup of coffee and have a think!

☺ . . . there are also a few of these. I'm not sure what they mean! I've put them in where there is a comment to make, something I agree with, or a good point – I think!

GLOSSARY

I know the glossary is usually at the back of normal books. Well, this is no ordinary book. The information you need to get the best out of the book is in the front.

Seems about right to me!

Put two lawyers together and they can talk for a week, and you won't understand a word. Put two docs together and it could be a month before you make sense of anything! Put a lawyer and a doc together and you get the language of contracting, that even to old NHS hands takes some explaining. Here's a glossary of some of the phrases we are all about to come to know and love in the lexicon of the new contract!

Achievement payments: These are payments according to the practice's achieved number of points in the quality and outcomes framework.

Additional services: These cover:
1   cervical screening
2   contraceptive services
3   vaccinations and immunisations
4   child health surveillance
5   maternity services excluding intra partum care (which will be an enhanced service)
6   the minor surgery procedures of curettage, cautery, cryocautery of warts and verrucae, and other skin lesions.

Aspiration payments: These will be made to practices and will constitute advance payments of a third of the points score to which a practice is aspiring in the voluntary quality and outcomes framework.

Barnett formula: The Barnett formula translates changes to certain public expenditure programmes in England (Great Britain in the case of Northern Ireland) into equivalent changes in the overall budgets of Scotland, Wales and Northern Ireland on the basis of population shares.

Carr-Hill allocation formula: This is a new GMS resource allocation formula and will provide the basis for allocating funds for global sum resources and for quality payments. It takes account of determinants of relative practice workload and costs.

Directed enhanced services: Enhanced services that are under national direction with national specifications and benchmark pricing which all PCOs must commission to cover their relevant population. These cover support services to staff and the public in respect of the care and treatment of patients who are violent, improved access, childhood vaccinations and immunisations, influenza immunisations, quality information preparation and advanced minor surgery.

Enhanced services: These are:

1 essential or additional services delivered to a higher specified standard, for example extended minor surgery

2 services not provided through essential or additional services. These might include more specialised services undertaken by GPs or nurses with special interests and allied health professionals and other services at the primary–secondary care interface. They may also include services addressing specific local health needs or requirements, and innovative services that are being piloted and evaluated.

Essential services: These cover:

1 the management of patients who are ill or believe themselves to be ill with conditions from which recovery is generally expected, for the duration of that condition, including relevant health promotion advice and referral as appropriate, reflecting patient choice wherever practicable

2 the general management of patients who are terminally ill

3 the management of chronic disease in the manner determined by the practice, in discussion with the patient.

Expert patient initiatives: Lay-led self-management training programmes for patients with some chronic diseases, encouraging effective self-management and better use of primary care and general practice by giving them greater knowledge of their condition so that they may improve their level of self-management and also help other patients.

Global sum: This money paid to practices includes provision for the delivery of essential and additional services, staff costs and locum reimbursement, including for appraisal, career development and protected time. It does not include money for various other items including: premises, IT, doctor-based payments, the equivalent of target payments, more advanced minor surgery and others.

Greenfield sites: An area, or areas, within a PCO that, due to a significant increase in the local population, requires the provision of new primary care services.

Gross Investment Guarantee: This ensures that the resources promised in this document will be delivered in aggregate. It includes money for the global sum, quality, transitional payments, premises and IT.

Guaranteed floor: A minimum, centrally specified amount of protected money from the PCO-controlled unified budget to ensure that there are sufficient funds for enhanced services.

Health Service Body: A body, such as a PCT in England, which can contract to provide NHS services under a NHS contract. It is expected that most practices would opt to become Health Service Bodies under the new GMS contract.

Holistic care payments: Paid to practices under the voluntary quality and outcomes framework for recognition of the breadth of achievement across the range of different clinical areas.

Independent contractor status: The method by which three quarters of all UK GPs contract with the NHS to provide services as self-employed independent contractors (see also *Salaried contractor*).

Local enhanced services: Enhanced services that are developed locally. The terms and conditions of these will be discussed and agreed locally between the PCO and the practice with, if wished, the involvement of the Local Medical Committee (LMC).

Market forces factor: Part of the methodology for calculating the global sum payment to practices. This factor takes into account the differential costs of the employment of practice staff throughout the UK.

National enhanced services: Enhanced services that have national specifications and benchmark pricing, but are not directed. These include intra partum care, anti-coagulant monitoring, intra-uterine contraceptive device fitting, more specialised drug and alcohol misuse services, more specialised sexual health services, more specialised depression services, multiple sclerosis, enhanced care of the terminally ill, enhanced care of the homeless, enhanced services for people with learning disabilities, immediate care and first response care and minor injury services.

NHS contract (in England): An arrangement under which one Health Service Body ('the acquirer') arranges for the provision to it by another Health Service Body ('the provider') of goods or services – section 4 of the National Health Service and Community Care Act 1990.

Patient Forum: In England, established by section 15 of the National Health Service Reform and Health Care Professions Act 2002, inter alia, to monitor and review the range and operation of services provided by, or under arrangements made by, the Primary Care Trust for which it is established.

Patient Services Guarantee: This will ensure that patients will continue to be offered at least the range of services that they currently receive under the existing contract, particularly in the case of patients whose practice has opted out of certain additional services.

Preparation payments: Preparation payments will be made to practices to aid their implementation of the quality and outcomes framework. These payments are not conditional on achievement but they will enable practices to collect initial data to establish their current position in the framework.

Primary care performer lists: The term for the new single list that will encompass the current three separate list arrangements for GPs: the medical list for principals, the supplementary list for non-principals and the forthcoming services list for PMS providers.

Primary care provider: The new definition of a GMS or PMS practice. A GMS contract is a contract between a PCO and a provider made up of one or more individuals, at least one of whom must be a GP, who act on their own behalf in their beneficial interest and not as representatives of commercial bodies.

Remedial notice: The notice served by the PCO on a provider concerning the action to be taken, where the PCO believes that a provider has failed to perform a service or is otherwise in breach of the contract. This would include failure to meet minimum standards in accordance with the provisions in the contract.

Quality practice payment: Paid to practices in recognition of the breadth of achievement across the organisational, additional services and patient experience domains of the quality and outcomes framework.

Salaried contractor: A GP who is employed by either a PCO or a practice under a nationally agreed model contract, with a salary within a range set by the Review Body.

Strategic Service Development Plan: The proposals containing the strategic plans of PCOs for health service development and capital investment, including the plans for premises development and enhanced services.

UK tariff: The nationally agreed percentage of a practice's global sum if it chooses to opt out of additional services or out-of-hours cover.

Unified budget: The discretionary health service budget allocated to PCOs centrally. This is separate from the global sum allocated to practices and quality payments, which are non-discretionary.

Got all that? I'll try and keep the rest in English!

Introduction

I've got to be honest, I am not a fan of the new contract. I wish the GPs had never voted for it. But in July 2003, they did, with a huge majority.

For: 25 359
Against: 6586

At the time, I said that the vote told me there are only 6586 GPs who understand patients, taxpayers, their role in history, trade unions and healthcare. They were the ones who said 'no'.

A bit strong I suppose. But I was cross. I'm a big fan of primary care.

For me the 'yes' vote meant: patients will register with a practice not a doctor; doctors can opt out of foundation services at the heart of personal intimacy and family life; content for these services is to be provided by 'the management'; the doctor–patient partnership is dead.

The doctors were tempted by a whacking pay rise and who can blame them. But a pay rise based on a formula that has been shown to be flawed and a quality system based on a points scoring scheme, dependent on an IT system yet to be shown functioning in an everyday environment. To be frank, I doubt but a few GPs actually sat down and read the 66 page proposal and umpteen annexes.

I said I thought the 'yes' vote meant they have been suckered by a trade union in decline, desperate for a victory after the debacle of the consultant's contract. For a while now, the BMA has been estranged from government and they bundled the vote through. The BMA actually placed adverts in the doctors' press that said: 'vote for less work, more pay and a better pension' (*British Medical Journal*, middle week of June 2003). To hell with the patients, then!

I said I thought it was a disaster.

Well, I got that off my chest and started to think about how to make it work and what it really means. It ain't gonna go away, so we'd best make the best of it. I hope this Tool Kit helps. Good luck! Let's roll up our sleeves and have a go!

Roy Lilley
September 2003

WHAT GOES AROUND, COMES AROUND . . .

We take a lot for granted. The NHS, with all its faults and foibles, remains hugely popular and most of us, in our lifetime, will have cause to be truly grateful that Aneurin Bevan had the vision and the courage to take on his doubters and detractors to make it happen. Back in 1948, when the NHS was going through its difficult birth-pangs, the very idea was hugely controversial. Indeed, the doctors' trade union, the British Medical Association, launched a £1 000 000 fighting fund to stop the idea dead in its tracks. History does not appear to record what happened to the money!

It is easy to forget, at its inception, that the NHS was simply the nationalisation of the healthcare facilities and systems that were around at the time. The existing infrastructure, a mixed economy of provision – the private hospitals, the charities and friendly society systems – were all drawn together under one umbrella and called the National Health Service. The doctors hated the idea. They did not want to lose their independence. Newspapers of the day quoted doctors as not wanting to become 'little more than servants'.

Indeed, as far back as 1946, the BMA secretary, Dr Charles Hill, asked the nation, on a Pathe News film shown in cinemas up and down the country, 'Do you want your doctor to be the State's doctor?'

Interesting really, since the new contract makes it impossible for an individual patient to register with an individual doctor. Patients will now register with a practice. It looks like the idea of '*your doctor*' has finally bit the dust!

Oh, and where, under the provisions of the contract, GPs want to withdraw from providing services, the PCOs will look to a mixed economy of providers to replace them.

Do you think we're making progress?

AND, AT NO EXTRA CHARGE . . .

The negotiations for the new GP contract were not the only argy-bargy going on in the summer of 2003. Whilst the GPs were cutting up rough and getting themselves into the mother-of-all-messes over their contract calculations, the hospital consultants were having a go too!

The consultants had broken the first rule of negotiation – always leave yourself somewhere to go. They didn't and painted themselves into a very awkward corner. They were offered a deal – it was recommended by the BMA negotiators – but the rank and file gave it a raspberry and turned it down. The BMA's head negotiator resigned, the government said there was no Plan B, it all got very sulky and no one was speaking to anyone.

It took the resignation of the then Secretary of State for Health, on entirely unrelated matters, to break the deadlock and leave an opportunity for his successor to step in and have a fresh go.

This is what they appear to have settled on. Looks like a score-draw to me.

Sticking point	Solution
An arcane issue around the guidance that dealt with non-emergency work during weekend mornings and evenings.	They settled on a new form of words: 'Consultants will have the right to refuse non-emergency work at such times. Should they do so, there will be no detriment in relation to pay, progression or any other matter.'
The consultants wanted more pay for evening and weekend work and what they call plain-time rates between 7am and 10pm, and including weekend mornings.	Bit of a result for the consultants – evening and weekend sessions have been reduced from 4 to 3 hours. Plain time from 7am to 7pm weekdays only.
All consultants are supposed to have a job plan. Research indicates a lot do not. Nevertheless, there was a long-standing argument over job plan appeals and who should hear them.	Three member appeals panels would include an independent member selected from a list approved by the StHA and the BMA, as well as representatives of the consultant and the employer. The Trust Board has the right to the final decision – *quite right, too!*

Sticking point	Solution
Increasing managerial control – yawn!	They settled on this form of words: 'The new arrangements are emphatically not intended to diminish professionalism or override clinical judgement.' *Meaningless?*
Consultants would have to do one or two extra NHS sessions before they could carry out private work and there was a sticking point over newly-qualified consultants' sessions before they could rush off and earn loadsa' money elsewhere.	Agreed: 'Where full-time consultants are working the equivalent of 11 or more programmed activities a week for the NHS and agree this should form part of their job plan, they would not have to offer any additional work for the NHS'. *Result – an away win for the Department of Health!*
New consultants would have to devote 8 sessions a week to direct clinical care; established consultants only have to do 7.	All consultants will have to do 7.5 sessions of direct clinical care. *Classic, cut-it-down-the-middle result. Not worth the argument in the first place.*
And, just for fun . . .	Consultants will get up to 2 extra days holiday a year! *Not a bad result when you think how short of doctors we are!*

Does it leave patients any better off?

ARE YOU READY FOR THIS?

The working document is called:

> Investing in General Practice
> The New General Medical Services Contract

You might want to go to the BMA website and download a copy of the complete document. If only to leave it perched conspicuously on the edge of your desk, to impress everyone.

Or perhaps reading through the 66 pages of closely typed grunge might be the kind of thing that turns you on!

Whatever, you can find it at: http://www.bma.org.uk. Click-through to /NewGMSContract. The document has eight sections and various annexes that deal with the calculation of formulae, explanation and examples. To make life simple I've used the sections as the chapter headings in the book.

Here we go . . .

If all goes according to plan, fingers crossed, lucky rabbit's foot in the pocket and the tooth fairy pays a visit, this is the timescale and the path to primary care paradise . . . .

20 June 2003: GPs vote to accept the contract.

23 June 2003: deadline for legislation to be put before Scottish Parliament.

June 2003 onwards: practices start to talk to PCOs about enhanced services, what they don't want to do and, generally, get their heads around what this is all going to look like.

Mid-July 2003: legislation poked into the existing Health and Social Care (Community Health and Standards) Bill, for England, Wales and Northern Ireland.

Summer 2003: funding provided to pay for the quality targets preparation work (expected to be paid quarterly, to ease practice cash-flow).

April 2004: the Queen does her stuff, the legislation is given approval and contracts are implemented in full.

31 December 2004: the final deadline for PCOs to take over out-of-hours responsibility of the GPs who don't want to do it.

Think Box

Has anyone noticed how close the vote was to missing the Parliamentary deadline? Looks to me like they had to get a 'yes' vote – there was no plan 'B'.

Investing in general practice

INVESTING IN GENERAL PRACTICE

SUMMARY OF CHANGES

You can speed-read through this bit. It is a sort of summary, bugle-blowing, blurb and a let-it-all-hang-out section. But it will make you look like you know something!

The new GMS contract will:

- provide new mechanisms to allow practices greater flexibility to determine the range of services GPs provide, including opting out of additional services and out-of-hours care
- reward practices for delivering clinical and organisational quality, through the evidence-based quality and outcomes framework which is in line with professional practice, and for improving the patient experience
- facilitate the modernisation of practice infrastructure including premises and IT
- support the development of best human resource management practice and help GPs achieve a better work/life balance, support the development of practice management, and recognise the different needs of GPs in different localities, including GPs in deprived communities and in rural and remote areas
- provide for unprecedented and guaranteed levels of investment through a Gross Investment Guarantee. The contract allocates resources on a more equitable basis and allows practice flexibility as to how these are deployed from the global sum.

Then there is a bit about the contract creating higher quality, empowering patients, simplifying the regulatory framework and making sure that soufflés never sink in the middle.

Got it? Of course you have. 'Nuff said, move on.

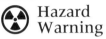 Hazard
Warning

Throughout the original document there is repeated reference to 'con-sultation'. It would be easy for 'consultation' to drift on and on and on and on and on and never reach a conclusion.

So, quite sensibly, all parties are committed to the Cabinet Office Code of Practice on Written Consultation, which sets out the arrangements and timescale for consultation *in normal circumstances*. This provides that, where consultation on written documents takes place, the period of consultation should normally last at least 12 weeks, other than in exceptional circumstances.

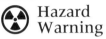 Hazard
Warning

Where services are being reconfigured or practices use their right to opt out of providing services, Primary Care Organisations (PCOs) will be responsible for ensuring that patient access to services is not compro-mised. Where practices opt out of services, their income (global sum) will be reduced and the PCO will be able to use this money to secure alternative provision from other practices or primary care providers, including PCOs themselves. This ignores the extra overhead costs the PCO is likely to incur.

The good or bad score card, the main changes at a glance:

	✔ Good	✗ Bad
1 Practices will be able to opt out of the provision of some services, either temporarily or permanently		
2 Patients will be registered with the practice and not the doctor		
3 GPs may no longer be responsible for out-of-hours care		
4 A new quality framework will reward practices for delivering quality care with extra incentives to encourage high standards		
5 Premises and IM&T will get more cash		
6 PCOs will fund the costs of practice IM&T systems, not the practice or the GP		
7 GPs will be able to move between salaried and independent contractor status		

	✓ Good	✗ Bad

8   The function of practice management will be enhanced, recognising the contribution an effective practice management can have in reducing the administrative burden on clinical staff

9   Practice managers will be encouraged to develop new roles and responsibilities following a new competency framework

10   Recognition of the special needs of the rural practice

11   A three year Gross Investment Guarantee which will be monitored by an independent Technical Steering Committee

12   The new Carr-Hill (some say Benny Hill!) allocation formula will provide equity, recognise case-mix and practice, when they can fine-tune it, make it work and sort it out

13   Funding will be provided irrespective of whether or not doctors are in place

14   A guaranteed floor of money from the unified budget of PCOs to ensure that enhanced services can be delivered where appropriate. This aims to help the shift of secondary care services into primary care

15   A new definition of pensionable pay with new flexibilities to facilitate portfolio careers

16   A Patient Services Guarantee, underpinned by the PCO

17   The new contract will normally be an NHS contract between the local Primary Care Organisation (PCO) and the practice, not the individual GP

18   In England and Wales, the existing three separate GP lists – the Medical List, the Supplementary List and the Services List – will be rationalised and replaced by a single Primary Care Performers List

19   *The Scottish Executive and the Northern Ireland Health Department will catch up and announce their respective plans for future listing arrangements in due course*

And, by the way, the new contract will be implemented in a phased way, allowing those elements that are not subject to primary legislation to be implemented more quickly. Substantial implementation will occur in 2003/04.

 Think Box

What's your score? Less than ten ticks and I'd say there's some serious thinking to do . . .

So you're going to be very busy!

MORE FLEXIBLE PROVISION OF SERVICES

Do you have problems with any of these issues?

	Yes	No
Poorly defined range of services		
Out-of-hours care		
Control of workload		
Insufficient resources		
Insufficient rewards		
Inhibited development of new services		
General practice an unattractive option for doctors		

If you do have problems, read on! There is good news. The contract deals with all these issues.

SERVICE CATEGORISATION

 Hazard Warning

PCOs are going to have a nice new job. It is their *statutory* duty to ensure patients can get access to the full range of primary medical services. Got that? *A statutory duty*. No messing. It's not down to the GPs anymore. It's a management job. Don't do it – go to jail!

WHAT SERVICES HAVE TO BE PROVIDED?

There are two Es and an Ooh! Essential services, enhanced services and out-of-hours services. However, it's not what you've got to do that's interesting. It's the bit that the docs don't have to do that is the most revealing . . .

THE FIRST E: ESSENTIAL SERVICES

- Services for patients who are ill or believe themselves to be ill, with conditions from which recovery is generally expected, for the duration of that condition, including relevant health promotion advice and referral as appropriate, reflecting patient choice wherever practicable.

> ☺ Patients who *believe themselves to be ill* – love that phrase!

- The general management of patients who are terminally ill.
- The management of chronic disease in the manner determined by the practice in discussion with the patient.

If that sounds like everybody, hold on. There is a whole list of stuff that is not considered 'essential':

- cervical screening
- contraceptive services
- vaccinations and immunisations
- child health surveillance
- maternity services – excluding intra partum care (which will be an enhanced service)
- the minor surgery procedures of curettage, cautery, cryocautery of warts and verrucae, and other skin lesions.

☀ Think
Box

Here's the question. Why wouldn't a GP want to do that sort of stuff? It seems to me it is at the very heart of family practice. Looking after kids and mums is what they do, isn't it?

If a practice opts out of providing this kind of service, the PCO has to step in and do it. What's the gold standard? I don't know. What I do know is, if the GPs don't want to do it, or can't do it, there'll be a reason.

Does it mean PCOs will be driven to cobble together a service out of a Portakabin on the other side of town and try and get all the immunisations and smears done at the same time? Does this mean harassed mums with two kids in a buggy will have to traipse, on a bus, in the rain, to get sorted? In those circumstances, my money says a lot won't bother and we could be in a real mess . . .

Here's the first job.

Who is going to decide if there are services in the opt-out that you don't want to do? What is the basis for the decision and do you want to be able to revisit it? How will you settle differences in view? And what planning is required to ensure that these services remain available to those who need them?

For example, childhood vaccination and immunisation schemes are additional services, and the infrastructure costs of delivering these have been built into the global sum paid to the practice. The financial incentives are high, but are they high enough to encourage high population coverage?

THE NEXT E: ENHANCED SERVICES

What are they? Here's the definition:

> 'Enhanced services are essential or additional services delivered
> to a higher specified standard, for example:
> • extended minor surgery
> • specialised services undertaken by GPs or nurses with special
>   interests *(include allied health professionals in your thinking)*
> • services at the primary care/secondary care interface
> • services addressing specific local health needs or requirements
> • innovative services that are being piloted and evaluated.'

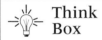 **Think Box**

Have you got any of these? GPs with a special interest, nurses running clinics, populations with special needs. Is this a good time to think about doing a health needs assessment or a practice audit, to figure out just what is being done, what could be done and what folk don't want to do any more?

This is important, as it will impact on the practice income at the one end, and at the other, the work of the PCO.

Time to think about leveraging up quality, or letting go . . . ?

Time to get organised.

THAT FORMULA!

Practice workload and the different groups of patients practices might be faced with, are part of the decision making process. The variation is recognised in the infamous Carr-Hill allocation formula, now known by some irreverent observers as the Benny Hill formula. Who, *Moi?* . . . No, no!

The idea was that the formula would determine the global sum payments, reflecting morbidity factors and the varying workload involved for practices in delivering care to very different groups of patients.

However, unless you've been in North Korea, or living down a hole in the ground, you will know that the poor old formula came in for a bit of a bashing when it was discovered that half of GP practices would be worse off under it. One thing that GPs are very good at is taking the back of an envelope and working out how much money they are going to make. And why not? They are self-employed and need to keep an eye on the cash.

So the formula has been parked, to be tinkered with and fiddled about with. The *BMA News* reported, 28 June 2003:

'Work starts to iron out flaws in formula and its funding'

Quite why a self-employed GP would vote for a new contract without really understanding how much he or she was going to get paid is a complete mystery to me. But what do I know, I've only been self-employed for 35 years!

There is going to be some sort of an enquiry to dig out what went wrong. I guess the answer is: someone lost the calculator . . .

Anyway, back in the real world, a Minimum Practice Guarantee makes sure that, in the short term, no one loses out and the GPs get their pay rise! The BMA say they are going to 'closely monitor' PCOs to ensure they spend their allocated budgets on enhanced services.

There doesn't seem to be any timescale for sorting this out . . .

HERE ARE THE IMPORTANT BITS FOR PCOS

The PCO can make more money available for enhanced services for particular groups of patients. For example, those who are difficult to manage *(I wonder if that means me? Yes – Ed)*. However, they can only do so after having funded up to the guaranteed minimum level of invest-ment. That was: £315/£394/£460m for 2003–2006 in England (HSC 2002/012).

✓ In case you were worrying: comparable funding will be made available in the other three countries. This freedom will subsume existing Local Development Schemes, the Improving Primary Care incentive scheme, services currently delivered under HSG(96)31, GPs with Special Interests (GPwSIs) and schemes to improve patient access. Existing contracts for such services will be rationalised into a single arrangement for enhanced services under the contract between the PCO and practice from 2004/05, and will continue for at least the duration agreed previously between the PCO and the practice – so no backsliding or reneging on deals!

But it has since been jacked up to £315/£518/£586m. There is a technical reason for this, to do with service categorisation, but unless you are a complete NHS anorak, we don't need to worry about that here!
By the way . . .

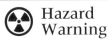 Hazard
Warning

The quality information preparation is important because a large part of the practice income is derived from quality payments. The scoring (dealt with later in the Tool Kit) depends on good information and IT. As many practices don't have the kit there is an interim, cobble-together solution. So pay attention!

The specifications for the directed and national enhanced services were published in the second contract document in May. They cover support services to staff and the public for the care and treatment of patients who are violent, improved access, childhood vaccinations and immunisations, flu immunisations, minor surgery *and for 2003/04 and 2004/05, quality information preparation.*

 Think
Box

Why are important foundation, family services such as childhood vaccinations and immunisations and flu immunisations 'enhanced'? They are bedrock? Aren't they? Apparently, it is because they are so important that they are separately incentivised in an effort to make it worthwhile for the GPs to do. The result? Better coverage. Do you buy that?

Other enhanced services have national minimum specifications and bench-mark pricing and include services not contained in the current GMS arrangements.

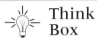 **Think Box**

Clever folk have been trying to shift services nearer to the patient, out of secondary care and into primary care, for as long as I can remember. The problem has included skills and premises, but mainly how to cover the running cost void, left in secondary care, when a lump of services are carved out. This might just be the answer?

Whaderyerfink?

This is the money that helps move some services from secondary into primary care. What does it include? Here's the list:

- intra partum care
- anti-coagulant monitoring
- providing near-patient testing
- intra-uterine contraceptive device fitting
- more specialised drug and alcohol misuse services
- specialised sexual health services
- specialised depression services
- more specialised services for patients with multiple sclerosis
- enhanced care of the terminally ill
- enhanced care of the homeless
- enhanced services for people with learning disabilities
- immediate care and first response care
- minor injury services.

Plus enhanced schemes may also be developed in response to local need, for which you have to work out terms and payments together, like grown-ups!

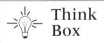 **Think Box**

Here's an interesting bit . . .

The PCO will also be able to provide the services itself. The practice is only a 'preferred supplier' and a PCO has the right to commission services, from another practice or an alternative provider, or do it itself.

Do you spot the sizzling bit? Isn't it burning off the page? Smokin'! The phrase 'An alternative provider'! Very significant.

> ☺ Does this mean a PCO could ask a drugs manufacturer to take on the care of a group of patients? Asthma, diabetes or blood pressure, for example? You bet it does. There's going to be some guidance issued that will deal with the possibility in more detail. But this is a definite 'watch this space' issue.

The approach is called disease management and has been around for ages. Indeed, the last guidance on the subject was Circular 94/94. It made disease management almost impossible to do.

That guidance has now expired and has not been replaced. So, the rules are – the old guidance pertains.

However, disease management, where a drugs or specialist firm is given the role of looking after (mainly chronic) conditions, is not uncommon in the USA. It is done against tight, quality-driven contracts that penalise the contractor for, for example, unplanned patient admissions into secondary care.

Who will be the first PCO to give it a try? Why not you?

Can you list the pros and cons?

It is a good idea because	It is a bad idea because

AND NOW THE OOH: THE BIG ONE!

Out-of-hours care

 This is going to need a bit of thought and several gallons of coffee, tea or something stronger . . .

There is a funny phrase that they use to describe the present situation. I think it's borrowed from the IT industry. Computer buffs will recognise it. Out-of-hours responsibility is described as follows:

the existing default responsibility is the GP's.

In plain English it means that out-of-hours services are down to the GPs. It seems to me the BMA thinks that, in large measure, the current dearth of GPs is because they have a 24-hours responsibility. The fact that most of them have already got it sorted seems to have escaped the big brains at the BMA.

☺ In case you were wondering, the term 'out-of-hours period' is defined as from 6.30 pm to 8 am on weekdays, and also the whole of weekends, Bank Holidays and public holidays.

So, there will be changes! Out-of-hours care will transfer to PCOs, who will become responsible for commissioning and, where necessary, providing the out-of-hours service. If practices want to carry on with their out-of-hours services, they can, but they will have to meet the PCO and national quality standards.

After 31 December 2004, it changes a bit. If, at that point, a practice decided it would take on an out-of-hours responsibility, they would be competing with other providers. So, no favours.

✓ There is nothing to stop practices providing surgeries for routine consultations in the evening or at weekends. It is paid for through the global sum unless you can persuade the PCO it is an enhanced service. So the trick seems to be to get loadsa patient support.

So, stuck with this responsibility, what does the PCO do and where do they go to for a service? Well, think laterally is the answer. Include:

• NHS Direct and NHS 24
• NHS walk-in centres
• GP cooperatives
• partnerships between practices
• GPs and primary care nurses in A&E departments
• community nursing teams
• commercial deputising services.

Not too lateral is it! All these great ideas are in the BMA documentation . . . Let's take a closer look at them.

What do you think will happen to the costs and quality of commercial deputising services if they suddenly find half the PCOs in the country knocking on their door, desperate for a solution to their out-of-hours problems?

NHS Direct and what-not is fine, provided the person at the call centre doesn't think you need to see a doctor. Walk-in centres only do very basic stuff. GP cooperatives are what we do now, as are partnerships between practices.

GPs in A&Es are OK if you don't mind adding to the numbers attending A&E. Community nursing teams will work for existing customers and commercial deputising services are already making a killing.

There is nothing new here and, in my view, nothing very helpful. It looks to me as though PCOs are likely to be up against it.

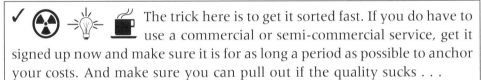 The trick here is to get it sorted fast. If you do have to use a commercial or semi-commercial service, get it signed up now and make sure it is for as long a period as possible to anchor your costs. And make sure you can pull out if the quality sucks . . .

This has to be done and dusted by New Year's Day 2004. Everyone will be doing it and my prediction is that the OOHs boys will think it's Christmas every day.

At the moment the price for an opt-out, for an average GP, is £6000. How long will it be before it's £8000? This has the potential to be a very cost-inflationary policy.

Don't get caught out. Have a good old think about this.

There are examples of innovative schemes (try the BMA website), and national teams of experts (via the Strategic Health Authority) will come and pay you a visit and help PCOs to develop new out-of-hours arrangements locally.

The problem with this is, no one is an expert. This is going from a cottage industry of solutions to a global whizz-bang, in the blinking of an eye.

And it gets worse!

 Hazard Warning

PCOs will be required to have a contingency plan in place which can be put into *immediate operation* should an out-of-hours provider fail.

Oh heck, how did the GPs get away with this? What to do?

Answer: get on with it!

And there is more. Just in case the PCOs were thinking of doing a bit of backsliding, until April 2004 out-of-hours will remain the responsibility of the individual GP.

Good news. However, between April 2004 and December 2004, out-of-hours will be a unique type of additional service and by 31 December 2004, all PCOs should have put in place effective alternative provision and have *taken full responsibility for out-of-hours*.

There will be a scramble for solutions. There are not enough deputising services, not enough GPs who will want to syndicate this and, frankly, the other ideas are %^&*, and are not going to solve the major problem.

> ✓ Another trick might be to work with other PCOs to find solutions and get a lever on cost and quality. If the PCOs stick together they could stop a Klondike – but for how long . . .

The ones that are left and willing to take on the job will name their price, go to work in a Ferrari and live in Monte Carlo for three months of the year.

Oh, and the final bad news is that those nice people from the Strategic Health Authorities will performance-manage this process.

> ☺ There is a ray of hope, but only if you live in the sticks. In remote and isolated areas, there may be no alternative to the present practice provision.

Sorry . . . it's a tough job and that's why you are so loved and rewarded for doing it! Thank you!

> ✓ **What to do?**
> This book is being written in July 2003. I make that about 360 working days until the deadline, at the end of December 2004, when the world becomes a more difficult place. By then PCOs will have to have both their new arrangements and their back-up in place.
> I guess by the time you get your hands on this book you could be looking at about 300 days, or maybe less.

✓ The favourite trick of the project planner is to start with a clean sheet of paper and write the end date at the bottom. At the top of the page write the current date. Measure off the working weeks and the days and write in review days and put in a false end date, to give yourself a bit of wriggle room at the end. The question then is simple: *'What do I have to be doing today to get to the end date, on time, project completed, the right way up, bright-eyed and bushy-tailed'?* It really is as simple as that.

But first . . . review the current out-of-hours arrangements. Can you continue to rely on them, or develop them? Will you have to start again?

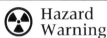 Hazard
Warning

One point cannot be stressed too much. There will be a scramble to get this sorted out and that means the potential for prices to go up!

Also, out-of-hours services will increasingly depend on locums and deputising services. There are issues of making sure these docs are appropriately qualified, up-to-date and aware of practice requirements, procedures, prescribing, access to notes, IT and all manner of tricky things.

✓ If you are hiring a deputising service, before granting them a contract, go out with them for a couple of nights, or weekends. See how they work. Will they do what you want them to do? Ring them at 3am and see what happens . . .

GET PLANNING NOW!

There are 6 'A's in success:

	Not done it	Doing it (by whom and when)	Done it
Audit – *what happens now?*			
Assess – *any good, lessons to learn?*			
Assemble – *new solution*			
Audit – *will it work?*			
Apply it – *get it in place early*			
Audit – *review, is it working?*			
Modifications?			

How do I get from here to there? Project planner:

Date	Where should I be today?	Done
Benchmark/review date		
Benchmark/review date		
Benchmark/review date		
False end date to allow for review		
End date	Complete	Paradise, Promotion, Prizes!

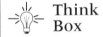 **Think Box**

There is nothing to stop a practice from opting out of out-of-hours responsibility and an individual member of the practice working a few weekends a month for a deputising service! Funny old world, ain't it?

OK, so you've got that sorted, here's a bit more to keep you awake at night.

IN-HOURS HOME VISITING SERVICES

If you work in a practice you have to write a practice leaflet, telling patients about when they can ask for a home visit!

Forget any idea of patients, customers, service and all that other good stuff that makes the world go around. This is the NHS. We tell our customers when they can be customers . . .

Under the new contract, patients are to be made aware of the new UK criteria for determining when home visits are necessary and these will be set out in the practice leaflet.

What goes in the leaflet? How about this for a start:

'. . . a practice will provide at the home of a registered or a non-registered patient in its practice area such services as the practice is contracted to provide during hours which do not fall in the out-of-hours period when, in light of the patient's medical condition, the doctor considers that such services are needed and would most appropriately be delivered by means of a home visit.'

Wise words according to the BMA

Very patient-friendly! Thank you. But, the curious thing is, you don't have to do in-hours home visits. If you want to become even further estranged from the idiosyncratic thought that family doctoring is about family doctoring, you can agree with the PCO for them to do it for you.

The PCO can, in agreement with local practices, invest in an area-wide home visiting service through the enhanced services scheme, to deliver services to patients that are less disruptive of daytime surgeries.

Just like the out-of-hours service. But in-hours, if you see what I mean! But it'll cost ya! It will follow a locally agreed transfer of resources. The PCOs can also provide transport to the surgery if they think it's 'desirable'.

 Hazard Warning

OK, so what happens if a patient reads the practice leaflet and decides not to call the doctor out, then becomes more sick, and dies?

 Hazard Warning

What happens if a patient calls for a visit and is told they don't meet the criteria – and they become more sick and die?

What happens in a part of town where there is a huge ethnic population? For example, in the area covered by the Homerton Hospital in East London, they translate their leaflets into 17 languages. Bear in mind that the NHS is only officially funded for translation of documents into Welsh. I suspect there are more Bangladeshi and Urdu speakers in the UK than there are Welsh speakers. So a patient never gets to read the patient leaflet in a language they can understand?

✓ Ask the UK's leading health risk management guru, Dr Paul Lambden, and he will tell you; *'Called out? When in doubt, go visit! The doctor has to make a judgement.'*

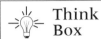

Think Box

This is a huge shift of responsibility to the PCO.

OH, NON-REGISTERED PATIENTS: BETTER NOT FORGET THEM . . .

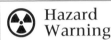

Hazard Warning

Have you got any good and accurate records for what happened in the last five years?

No change here. The obligation to provide immediate/necessary/emergency treatment and treatment to temporary residents will remain. There will be a simplified payment method by a single allocation included within the total funding arrangements, called the Global Sum. This will be calculated on the basis of the average number of claims in the practice over the previous five years.

If you are getting more than your share of non-reg patients, now is the time to make changes. You can agree with the PCO to fund it as an enhanced service.

NON-NHS WORK

Yes, we all know the proper role of the GP is the care of patients *who are or believe themselves to be ill* – I love that phrase! – but we also know that in the real world docs end up writing medical reports and what-not.

New arrangements will let you charge for:

- examining *(but not treating)* a patient for a report on injuries sustained in a road traffic accident or a criminal assault
- providing drugs and/or medical supplies, including travel kits, which a patient requires while he or she is abroad *(this is in addition to existing provisions in respect of travel vaccines)*

- attending and examining *(but not treating)* a patient at the request of a commercial, educational or not-for-profit organisation for the purpose of writing a medical report or certificate
- attending and examining *(but not treating)* a patient for the purpose of writing a medical report required in connection with a claim for compensation against any public or private body
- examining *(but not treating)* a patient for the purpose of writing a 'fit to travel by air' report.

YOU DON'T HAVE TO DO IT . . . .

OPTING OUT OF ADDITIONAL SERVICES

Too busy, can't get the staff? There's stuff you can opt out of.
   Let's start with temporary opt-outs. These might be:

- the practice has never provided the service
- no one to do it, lack of skills within the practice
- conscientious grounds
- opted-out more than twice in three years with no sign of a solution.

> ✓ The first step is to get talking, find a solution.

The first time around, the PCO and the practice should try and resolve the issue. When a practice wants to opt out it must give notice to the PCO, with their reasons. However, if a practice is providing any enhanced service(s), or any additional services to patients of another practice, the PCO may refuse to accept notice.
   If the talking fails, the practice must confirm to the PCO its intention to withdraw from the provision of a service and whether this is a temporary (less than a year) or a permanent withdrawal.

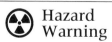 **Hazard Warning**
This is coming at PCO management very fast – are they ready for this?

PERMANENT WITHDRAWAL

Preparations for opting out commenced from April 2003 and the first withdrawals can occur from April 2004.

Meanwhile, practices facing workload or workforce pressures can talk with their PCO about how to solve the problems, including what support the PCO can provide.

✓ PCOs need to find out, during the 2003/04 contracting round, about any potential withdrawals or intention to provide additional or enhanced services not currently delivered.

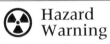 **Hazard Warning**

Let's not forget the punter. Consultation with affected patients should be carried out as quickly as possible and should not be a reason to delay implementation of the opt-out.

TEMPORARY OPT-OUT: HERE ARE THE RULES

- PCOs to agree the opt-out as quickly as possible given the immediate nature of the problem *(don't wait for the more time-consuming rules for permanent opt-out)*.

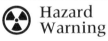 **Hazard Warning**

Informing patients of a temporary transfer of services? Is a poster in the practice waiting room good enough, or is this a leaflet job? Ad in the local paper? Round-robin letter? Or what? Phone call? Visit?

- Opt-out to be for a minimum period of six months and a maximum of 12 months (more than 12 months will normally constitute a permanent opt-out), but the PCO has the flexibility to agree more in exceptional circumstances.
- Practices and PCOs will be required to agree how best to inform patients of a temporary transfer of the service.

- PCOs will, where appropriate, agree with the original provider a programme of development, training or support in readiness for re-provision, where these were factors in the original decision to opt out.

> ✓ The money? The PCO will recoup a UK-wide fixed cost for the service (weighted according to the Carr-Hill formula) and the practice budget will be reduced by this amount.

THE WAY BACK?

Progress towards re-provision will be reviewed. If the PCO:

- agrees that the practice is able to re-provide the service, the service will revert back to the original provider at the agreed date
- does not consider the practice is able to provide the service within the agreed timescale, it can inform the practice of its intention to seek an alternative provider and follow the normal procedures for permanent opt-out.

> ✓ In some circumstances where the practice is unable to resume, it could be due to factors outside their control, in which case the PCO has discretion to extend the length of temporary withdrawal.

TEMPORARY BECOMES PERMANENT

If the practice wants a permanent opt-out they have to inform the PCO *as soon as possible* and *not later than three months* before the agreed re-provision date.

Oooh, wet towel time for the PCO. They are responsible for sorting out the alternative services.

> 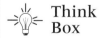 **Think Box**
>
> Doesn't this all seem a bit one-sided? The poor old PCO could be stuck with a real mess? If the practices don't want to do something you can bet that, nine times out of ten, there will be a logistical or staffing problem. Shuffling it over to the PCO doesn't strike me as a solution.

PERMANENT OPT-OUT

Here are the rules:

- The practice gives three or six months' notice of its wish to opt out permanently.

 Think Box

How good is this for patients? Where alternative provision has not been secured after six months there will be a further and final three month transitional period. At this stage the PCO and practice will discuss and agree effective local mechanisms for providing the service until such a time as alternative provision is in place, but for not longer than three months.

- During which time it is starting to look as if the patient will have to put up with an indifferent service, run by people who'd rather be doing something else. Tell me I'm wrong – please!
- Where necessary, the PCO will notify the practice at two months that the practice is required to continue provision for six months in total.
- The practice and PCO will be required to agree how best to inform affected patients *(Mmmm – see previous Hazard Box on the topic)*.
- The PCO will become responsible for providing the service after nine months.

This depends on a lot of talking, agreement and touchy-feely, woolly stuff. If it gets rancorous – and who is going to argue that there isn't huge potential for that – what happens? Does anyone want to bet that opting-out isn't going to become a bargaining chip in the game of 'gimme-more-resources'.

When all else fails, in steps the Strategic Health Authority, who will pronounce the wisdom of Solomon, or put the boot in, to resolve it.

IN, OUT, IN, OUT, SHAKE IT ALL ABOUT . . .

When a practice opts out of a service on a permanent basis, it cannot seek to re-provide it until the contract with the alternative provider ends. And, by the way, the rules of open competition would then apply.

PERHAPS IT'S NOT ALL ONE-SIDED

NEW ABILITY FOR PCOS TO PROVIDE OR COMMISSION CARE

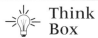 **Think Box**

At your next meeting, you can drop this into the conversation: out goes the old section 56 of the National Health Service Act 1977 and a chunk of section 33 of the National Health Service (Scotland) Act 1978 and Article 51 of the Health and Personal Social Services (NI) Order 1972.

There is a new trick called the Patient Services Guarantee *(of which more later – see page 104)*. The PCOs have to ensure they are delivering it. If they are not, they can provide the services themselves or commission them from alternative providers.

When a practice wants to withdraw from an additional service, the PCO can go shopping to ensure the effective alternative provision of services:

- from another practice that is normally providing the full range of additional services to its own registered patients and has an open list
- from 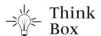 an alternative provider
- by providing the service itself.

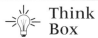 **Think Box**

An 'alternative provider'? Very interesting. From the private sector? Why not. From a pharmaceutical company perhaps, or even Johnny Foreigner! Wow, exciting time coming. Look out for more guidance . . .

☺ There is a little-noticed facility in the contract for practices to delegate services to other providers, with no loss of quality points.

There'll be all sorts of caveats about cost and quality, but it's an interesting direction of travel.

At a time when the NHS has too many customers, docs and nurses in short supply, a shake-up of provision and a mixed economy of providers is the ineluctable next step.

PCOs will be able to:

- provide additional or enhanced services if they are able to offer the same or better value for money, or the same or higher standards of care for patients than other interested parties
- offer support to practices to enable them to maintain their provision of additional services rather than have to withdraw as a first option.

Including:

- maintaining a range of full-time or part-time salaried staff *(clinical and non-clinical)*
- buying contracted sessions, as and when required, from existing practice-based staff on an ad hoc basis, in agreement with their employers
- commissioning services from an alternative provider
- making an agreement with doctors as a means of creating a bank of local support.

> This all looks like fun and a very different NHS. What do you think? Will PCOs use their powers rarely, to trim services; quite often, to keep them going; or seriously, to change the face of primary care?

Never mind the quality, feel the width

NEVER MIND THE QUALITY, FEEL THE WIDTH

REWARDING QUALITY AND OUTCOMES

I've never really understood the NHS's attitude to quality. In the real world, outside the NHS, quality is the foundation of everything. No quality, no business. End of story. It is not an add-on, a bolt-on or an extra. Quality is what underpins the organisation. The reward for quality is customers.

In the NHS, quality is seen as something different. It has become an add-on. Services keep going, quality or not. And quality is rewarded. So half-good quality gets half the reward. Sadly, I don't think this contract does much to drag the NHS into the real world where quality is the baseline.

The BMA contract document says this:

> 'Practices already provide a quality service, although the existing GMS contract places far greater emphasis on high volume than quality of care. Less than 4 per cent of the total current spend on fees and allowances is explicitly derived from quality of care. This emphasis runs counter to GPs' professionalism, the interests of the NHS, and the interests of patients.'

Well, do they? Do practices 'already provide a quality service'? Some do, but for sure some don't. Can we have volume and quality? The car industry seems to manage it. Yes, I know, before you reach for your pen and write to me; healthcare is not car making. But there has to be a parallel. Why else would there be a debate around NHS quality at all? The NHS has to learn to do volume without sacrificing quality.

The new contract introduces a quality and outcomes framework. They are so keen on quality they are even going to pay for it before they get it. Payments to prepare for entering the quality and outcomes framework will be guaranteed to all practices in 2003/04. Thereafter, there is a lot more money on offer.

WHAT'S IN THE NEW QUALITY FRAMEWORK?

Well, we start with a new word in the lexicon of healthcare:

Domains

The framework is full of **domains** and each domain contains a range of **areas** described by key **indicators**.

Got that? Domains, areas and key indicators. Drop those words into a conversation and you'll sound like you know something!

There are four domains:

* clinical
* organisational
* additional services
* patient experience.

CLINICAL DOMAIN

This contains ten disease areas:

* asthma
* cancer
* chronic obstructive pulmonary disease (COPD)
* coronary heart disease (CHD) including left ventricular dysfunction (LVD)
* diabetes
* epilepsy
* hypertension
* hypothyroidism
* mental health
* stroke and transient ischaemic attacks (TIA).

There is no point in reproducing all the quality indicators here as they are available in guidance, on the BMA website, the chip-shop and just about everywhere. However, here's an example of what to expect:

Secondary prevention in Coronary Heart Disease – Summary of points
All minimum thresholds are 25%

Indicator	Points	Maximum threshold
Medical records		
CHD 1. The practice can produce a register of patients with coronary heart disease	6	
Diagnosis and initial management		
CHD 2. The percentage of patients with newly diagnosed angina (diagnosed after 1 April 2003) who are referred for exercise testing and/or specialist assessment	7	90%
Ongoing management		
CHD 3. The percentage of patients with coronary heart disease, whose notes record smoking status in the past 15 months, except those who have never smoked, where smoking status need be recorded only once	7	90%
CHD 4. The percentage of patients with coronary heart disease who smoke, whose notes contain a record that smoking cessation advice has been offered within the last 15 months	4	90%
CHD 5. The percentage of patients with coronary heart disease whose notes have a record of blood pressure in the previous 15 months	7	90%
CHD 6. The percentage of patients with coronary heart disease, in whom the last blood pressure reading (measured in the last 15 months) is 150/90 or less	19	70%
CHD 7. The percentage of patients with coronary heart disease whose notes have a record of total cholesterol in the previous 15 months	7	90%
CHD 8. The percentage of patients with coronary heart disease whose last measured total cholesterol (measured in the last 15 months) is 5 mmol/l or less	16	60%
CHD 9. The percentage of patients with coronary heart disease with a record in the last 15 months that aspirin, an alternative anti-platelet therapy, or an anti-coagulant is being taken (unless a contraindication or side-effects are recorded)	7	90%
CHD 10. The percentage of patients with coronary heart disease who are currently treated with a beta blocker (unless a contraindication or side-effects are recorded)	7	50%
CHD 11. The percentage of patients with a history of myocardial infarction (diagnosed after 1 April 2003) who are currently treated with an ACE inhibitor	7	70%

. . . are you starting to get a feel for what is happening?

The idea is that the practice has a look at the indicators and makes a decision. How much of the target to go for? All of it, 100%, or 30% (the minimum is 25%)?

✓ For example, how many of your CHD patients have notes that, in the last 15 months, record if they are a smoker? Apart from the ones who have never smoked, that is. If the answer is all of them, you can commit to the top end, 90% target and collect seven quality points.

And we know what points mean! *(Yes, thank you – Ed)* Well, points mean prizes, or in this case, cash.

✓ If you've got all of your appropriate CHD patients on aspirin, an alternative anti-platelet therapy, or an anti-coagulant – collect another seven points.

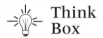 **Think Box**

So, here's the question: how are you going to decide what percentage of the target to go for?

✓ Design some audit methodology to assess what targets the practice should aim for. Do not leave it for the one who shouts the loudest to make the decision. If you guess, you'll get it wrong, look stupid and it could end up costing you money because if you don't hit what you commit to, they can rake the money back.

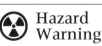 **Hazard Warning**

Bear in mind that this is a year-on-year indicator. You might think it's worth starting at the low end of what you know you can do and advance from there.

If you've got at least 60% of your CHD patients with a measured cholesterol of 5 mmol/l (measured in the last 15 months), collect a big win bonus of 16 points.

ORGANISATIONAL DOMAIN

This contains five areas:

- clinical and practice management
- communicating with patients
- education and training
- medicines management
- records and information.

ADDITIONAL SERVICES DOMAIN

This has four areas:

- cervical screening
- child health surveillance
- contraceptive services
- maternity services.

PATIENT EXPERIENCE DOMAIN

Looks like they ran out of ideas here, there are only two areas:

- patient survey
- consultation length.

The BMA claims the indicators were 'developed by an expert group'. Well, rather a lot of the material appears to have come from the Royal College of General Practitioners' Quality Team Development and Practice Accreditation Scheme.

> 'The inclusion of patient experience in the quality framework of the new contract represents an opportunity', claims the BMA, 'for practices to obtain systematic feedback from their patients about the services they provide and how they are provided, and to include these in their service development plans as well as engaging patients in service redesign.'

Call me a hard-faced unreconstructed old cynic, but aren't many practices already doing this? And there are a number of patient questionnaires in existence. Have they changed anything?

Do you know anything about patient experiences being changed? Let me know if you do!

How hard is it to harvest a shedload of patient experience (PE) points? Here's the formula:

PE 1 Length of Consultations

The length of routine booked appointments with the doctors in the practice is not less than 10 minutes. [If the practice routinely sees extras during booked surgeries, then the average booked consultation length should allow for the average number of extras seen in a surgery session. If the extras are seen at the end, then it is not necessary to make this adjustment.]

For practices with only an open surgery system, the average face to face time spent by the GP with the patient is at least 8 minutes.

Practices that routinely operate a mixed economy of booked and open surgeries should report on both criteria.

30 points

PE 2 Patient Surveys

The practice will have undertaken an approved patient survey each year.

40 points

PE 3 Patient Survey

The practice will have undertaken a patient survey each year, have reflected on the results and have proposed changes if appropriate.

15 points

PE 4 Patient Surveys

The practice will have undertaken a patient survey each year and discussed the results as a team and with either a patient group or Non-Executive Director of the PCO. Appropriate changes will have been proposed with some evidence that the changes have been enacted.

15 points

There is little doubt that some practices will struggle on the 10 minute per consultation target. However, as it is almost impossible to audit, perhaps they'll collect the points anyway *(Misanthropist – Ed)*.

Forty points for the patient survey? Easy, get a helpful pharma-rep to sort it out for you. There are two questionnaires that have been accredited. One is the Improving Patient Questionnaire (IPQ) developed by Exeter University and the other is the General Practice Assessment Questionnaire (GPAQ), developed by the National Primary Care Research and Development Centre in Manchester.

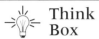

Think Box

The good old NHS has had to put up with naming and shaming. There is a new twist on this. It's called:

Gaming and not being ashamed!

Here's the trick. Ask yourself: is the aggravation and cost of going for a target outweighed by the financial reward? It may not be. And there is no obligatory threshold. If the practice doesn't want to play, then they don't play though they may earn less. There is no doubt that a careful analysis of the targets, measured against the practice profile, and performance will pay dividends. That's why practices need good practice managers!

LET'S GET DOWN TO THE DOSH!

It's easy to forget that the majority of primary care is delivered by self-employed practitioners. When they get paid, how they get paid and how much they get paid is very important to them!

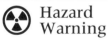

Hazard Warning

... practice managers will have to be really cute about managing finances, keeping on top of performance and payments. Otherwise they could end up with year-end problems.

The new deal places great emphasis on payments for quality. Quality can only be assessed after the event, so payments are retrospective – too retrospective and, just like any other small business, the practice has a cash flow problem and goes broke.

This is recognised in the contract and some payments are up front with a year-end adjustment. Nevertheless, practice managers will have to be really cute about managing finances, keeping on top of performance and payments. Otherwise they could end up with year-end problems.

Making payments

There are three types of payment:

- preparation payments (these are for the first two years only)
- aspiration payments (including additional infrastructure costs but not premises and IT)
- achievement payments.

 OK, make a coffee and let's see what this is all about . . .

Preparation payments – unkindly known by some acerbic gurus as money for nothing! *(Tut tut – Ed)*

Here's the situation. Big chunks of payments under the new contract are for quality. It is based on a point-scoring framework that has two distinct disadvantages.

- It's new and will take time to sort out, get in place, implement and all that other stuff. But there's no time to trial it, or test run it. It's got to go live.
- To make the system work properly a really super-duper IT system is needed – the problem is, many practices don't have the IT kit to do the job.

. . . So this time around the scheme is based on hit, hope, honesty and finding a four-leaf clover. Gimme strength!

Substantial quality preparation payments will be made in 2003/04 and 2005/06. You don't have to do anything to get these payments! (Who negotiated this?) Yup, these payments are not conditional on achievement *but they will enable practices to collect initial data to establish their current position in the framework.*

 Hazard Warning
How important is this to practice income? There are no words to describe the pivotal, essential, key, crucial and fundamental importance of getting this right.

This will tell you where to pitch your aspirational payment in the following year. They are not based on the Benny-Hill formula *(stop doing that – Ed)*, but on registered lists – and from 2003/04 they amount to an average of £9000 per practice in each of the three years.

To sort out the cash flow problems that annual payments might cause, they will be paid at the beginning of the financial year. Up front.

Aspiration payments – or 'keep yer fingers crossed' payments . . .

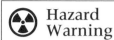 **Hazard Warning**

Good financial management is vital. Whatever practice budgets have looked like before, tear them up. You will have to get into zero-based budgeting and you may have to reschedule some payments or even revisit your facility with the bank.

From 2004/05, practices will agree their aspiration levels with PCOs and aspiration payments will be paid monthly alongside the global sum. Again, this helps to take the pressure off the cash flow and keep the bank manager happy. Even so, these payments will only be a third of the predicted total points, so cash flow management could be tight.

HERE'S THE FINGERS CROSSED BIT . . .

Even if the practice thinks it is only scoring a relatively low number of points in 2003/04, it will be free to aim as high as it wishes provided it can demonstrate to the PCO that it has a *reasonable* chance of achievement.

Get it? *Reasonable* chance. That's all, *reasonable* chance.

✔ So, for example, if an average practice which thinks it is scoring about 300 points in total across the framework in 2003/04 is aspiring to 750 points in 2004/05, it would receive an 'aspiration' payment for 250 points during 2004/05.

Achievement payments – or 'show me the beef' payments!

Achievement for 2004/05 will then be measured at the beginning of the following year, starting from 2005/06, and an achievement payment will be made. If you thought you'd achieve 750 points in 2004/05, you would receive an achievement payment for the remaining 500 points. However, as there will be no cap on quality, if the practice performed better than expected and achieved 900 points it would receive 650 points as its achievement payment, irrespective of the number of points it aspired to.

☢ Hazard Warning

Now here's the rub! This is the tricky bit and the bit that might send you begging to the bank – if the practice did not perform as well as expected and only achieved 400 points, it would only receive a further 150 points as its achievement payment.

Get it really wrong, achieve less than a third of your aspiration points, and the overpayment will be deducted from the aspiration payment for the following year.

Clearly, the big brains that negotiated this piece of multifarious wisdom thought you'd have to be a real bozo not to be able to turn in a third of your prediction – but you never know. Take nothing for granted and have a contingency in place in case the worst happened.

💡 Think Box

Now, forgive me if I am a touch cynical for a moment or two. None of this really works without the right computer software to make the achievements and points jump off the screen. Doing this job by hand is not an option. So here's the good news. Computer software will be provided in 2003/04 to all practices to enable them to calculate, at any point in time, what they are achieving.

Now, what do we know about computer software? I know what you're thinking. I've written it at the bottom of this box!

So keeping records, getting on top of computing and tight budget management is the new order of the day.

It never works first time around.

So you can see why I keep banging on about good financial planning and management.

At the beginning of 2005/06, the practice will also set out what it is aspiring to in that year, and similarly receive payment for a third of the points for that aspiration during the year, alongside the achievement payment for 2004/05.

How is this all calculated? Like I said, points mean prizes . . .

A practice's entitlement to quality payments will be determined through a quality scorecard, which assigns up to 1000 points for achievement and 50 points for maintaining improved access. Got that? Good. The BMA, in selling the deal to the docs, said: 'the quality scorecard was based on a desire for:

• simplicity
• transparency
• voluntarism
• continuous improvement
• rewarding breadth of service provision as well as depth
• minimising perverse incentives.'

They also said it was of a 'pioneering nature'! You can say that again! They know they are batting on what could be a very sticky wicket beyond 2005/06, so it may be adjusted in the, wait for it, 'light of lessons arising from its practical application in consultation and negotiation with the GPC'. Ho, ho! This is the get-out-of-jail condition in the contract! Nice one!

   Remember this: in 2004/05, based on current average list size, each point will be worth £75 per practice with an average weighted population. In 2005/06, it gets serious and the figure will rise to £120.

✓ To calculate your practice entitlement, multiply the number of points aspired to by the cash values of each point. This sum will then need to be multiplied by the ratio between the weighted practice population and the average weighted population. *Initial estimated weighted practice populations are yet to be announced and these will be sent direct to practices.* The practice entitlement will also depend on disease prevalence. The details of the calculation have yet to be agreed.

Clear as mud!

☼ ☺ ✓ On the BMA website you will find a really useful 'calcu-
lator' based on a Microsoft Excel spreadsheet that you can download and use to calculate your likely practice earnings.
   There was no point in printing it in a book as it is a 'live' document. It is worth a visit. Go to http://www.bma.org.uk, then click through to /NewGMSContract.

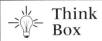 **Think Box**

Here's a thought: in line with the Gross Investment Guarantee, if there is an overall underspend on quality, the pounds per point could increase. So that means if enough practices screw up there might be more money for you! Pity the patients though, eh?

The practice will have complete freedom to choose which areas of the quality framework to focus on. All or nothing, it's up to you.

Oh, and don't forget that practices will also be eligible for holistic care and quality practice payments.

Here's the 2004/05 quality scorecard:

CHD including LVD, etc.	121	
Stroke or transient ischaemic attack	31	
Cancer	12	
Hypothyroidism	8	
Diabetes	99	
Hypertension	105	
Mental health	41	
Asthma	72	
COPD	45	
Epilepsy	16	
		Clinical maximum 550
Organisational indicators		
Records and information	85	
Patient communication	8	
Education and training	29	
Practice management	20	
Medicines management	42	
		Organisational indicators maximum 184
Additional services		
Cervical screening	22	
Child health surveillance	6	
Maternity services	6	
Contraceptive services	2	
		Additional services maximum 36
Patient experience		
Patient survey	70	
Consultation length	30	
		Patient experience maximum 100
Holistic care payments	100	
Quality practice payments	30	

To save you reaching for the calculator, the total for clinical, organisational, additional, patient experience, holistic care and quality service is a nice round 1000, with an extra 50, for the access bonus.

Total: 1050

HOW ARE POINTS SCORED?

Points are awarded for depth of quality in particular areas and breadth of achievement across the framework.
   Here's what the BMA says:

> 'To score points for the process and outcome indicators in a particular clinical area, a practice must have first achieved the structure indicator. Reflecting the key principle of voluntarism whereby clinicians may choose where to focus their energies, achievement against each indicator gives a points score which differs according to the associated workload. Achievement for each process and outcome indicator in the clinical areas is assessed by a percentage. A proportion of the points score for each indicator will be awarded in a direct linear relationship for achievement between the minimum, set at 25 per cent for the clinical indicators, and the maximum set for each indicator based on the evidence for the maximum practically achievable level to deliver clinical effectiveness.'

Errr, got that?

✓ Let's try an example:
   If 15 points were available for an indicator with a maximum level of achievement of 85% and the practice had achieved 65%, they would receive 40/60ths of 15 points, i.e. 10 points. Ugh!

It's easier to reckon up points for the organisational domain and additional services domain *(with the exception of the indicator for cervical screening coverage)* and patient experience domain; it's based on a yes, or a no!
   Thank goodness something's simple.

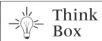 **Think Box**

Quite what, in the long run, this will do for patients, I'm not too sure. GPs can pull out of out-of-hours, day visits, pick and choose services and quality thresholds. This doesn't sound like much of a contract to me.

And there's more. If the patients get difficult, the practice doesn't suffer.

Practices will be able to exclude certain categories of patients from the calculation of performance, for example:

- patients who have been recorded as refusing to attend review and who have been invited on at least three occasions
- patients newly diagnosed within the practice or who have been newly registered with the practice, who should have measurements made within three months and delivery of clinical standards within nine months, for example lowering of cholesterol or blood pressure
- patients for whom it is not clinically appropriate, for example those who have an allergy, and other contraindications or adverse reactions, and the terminally ill
- where a patient has given informed dissent to treatment and this has been recorded in the records
- where a patient has not tolerated relevant medication
- patients who are on maximum tolerated doses of medication whose levels remain suboptimal
- where a patient has a supervening condition that makes treatment of their condition inappropriate, for example cholesterol reduction where the patient has liver disease.

Given the NHS's ability to fiddle figures, I can't wait to see what happens next! The PCO is supposed to be on the look-out for unexplained variances between the practice disease register and the overall level of morbidity within the PCO. Expect another three tonnes of guidance and targets to avalanche onto someone's desk. Let's hope it's not yours!

If the PCO thinks the practice is on the fiddle, making out that their failure to hit targets is all the fault of the nasty patients, they can consult with the Local Medical Committee. Then it gets complicated. The practice will be able to rescore the clinical achievement payments on the basis of an adjusted disease register reflecting average PCO morbidity.

The practice will have a right of appeal against such a decision.

Can you measure quality? Yup, you can measure anything!

Measuring breadth of quality

According to the BMA, they want to support the intrinsic nature of general practice. So they persuaded the negotiators to drop in a nice little earner. It's called the holistic care payment and will 'recognise breadth of achievement across the range of different clinical areas'.

How is it calculated? Oh, you'll love this:

> 'The scale of the holistic care payment is calculated by considering the proportion of points achieved in each of the 10 clinical areas. The proportion of points achieved for the third lowest clinical area determines the proportion scored of the total holistic care points available.'

✓ OK, let's try an example:

If a practice achieves half of the total number of points available in five clinical areas, a third in two, a quarter in another and nothing in the remaining two, the practice will be eligible for one quarter of the total holistic care payment.

The same approach applies for quality practice payments, which span all the areas within the organisational, additional services and patient experience domains.

And access? Well, for a lot of working folk, when they go to work in the morning, the practice is closed. When they come home in the evening, it is closed. On a Saturday it is open for emergencies and on a Sunday it is closed.

So, in recognition of the increase in workload required to deliver good access at the same time as higher quality, practices will be rewarded by a 50 points bonus score if they are achieving the relevant target.

Recording and reviewing arrangements

How else to measure achievements other than by relying on high quality information being available from the practice clinical systems? To qualify for payment, quality framework data will be recordable, repeatable, reliable, consistent and auditable.

That can't be done without IM&T systems. Apparently the Gods of Whitehall think it is a good idea for the taxpayer to train the staff to get the information from a system funded by the taxpayer, to calculate how much of the taxpayer's money will be spent rewarding self-employed contractors! *(Oh, too cynical – Ed.)* Sorry!

Education and training of practice staff will be supported through funded national programmes. UK-wide reporting queries will be developed, the GPC will be fully involved in defining these to meet the requirements of the quality framework, and software will be provided to all practices to enable them to calculate how their points will translate into rewards.

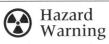 **Hazard Warning**

In the meantime, what happens? Well, by all accounts we are to trust practices to tell us . . . Personally, I don't find that very business-like. But what do I know?

In the words of the BMA:

> 'The practice quality review will be founded on the development of a relationship between the practice and the PCO based on the principles of high trust, evidence base, appropriate progression and development within the practice context, minimising bureaucracy, and ensuring compliance with the statutory responsibilities of the PCO.'

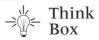 **Think Box**

Write down, here, what you'd do if someone, more senior than you, asked you to cheat . . .

  Sooner or later it will happen, if not to you, then to some poor soul.

The PCOs have a big role here. In the official phrase, *underpinned by statute* – which is to say, by law – the PCO's job is to get this lot sorted:

- Achievement against the quality framework will be reviewed by the practice providing annual information on its performance.
- The PCO will carry out visits to the practice annually.
- The evidence-based review will be against the agreed national standards set out in the quality and outcomes framework.
- The practice will submit a single standard return form, *which is being developed by the NHSC and GPC* and which cannot be extended locally.
- It will be used for practices to self-evaluate their performance and to provide evidence to substantiate their achievement of the quality standards.
- Each PCO visit will include a comprehensive review and discussion with clinicians and the practice manager.
- The visit will avoid disruption to patients or other members of the practice. The LMC may be involved in this process at the discretion of either party. The practice costs of preparation for the visit are built into the aspiration element of payments.

And . . .

- The frequency of visits may increase and additional supporting evidence may be required where there is concern around, for example, inaccurate practice information or suspected fraud.
- Participation in and approval through an accredited organisational quality programme can count towards points on the organisational domain.
- Existing schemes will be accredited for use in this way, and as a result validated achievement against relevant indicators will be subject to lighter touch monitoring as part of the annual review.

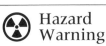 Hazard
Warning

If all is hunky-dory and the practice gets ticks in all the right boxes, the PCO will confirm the level of achievement funding to be paid. That's the time when the practice will also discuss the points to which it is aspiring in the following year.

There is a big impact on the annual planning cycle. The practice should be thinking, very early on in the year, where it intends to aim for in the following year. Not only is there an impact on financial planning and the funding of the practice activities, there could well be workforce issues. If you want to do something new, different, sexy and interesting, can you advertise for/recruit/train and get the staff you want, on board, in time?

Remember, good staff are probably already doing a good job for someone else. Getting staff decoupled from one employer and doing something really useful for you can take two to three months!

If it goes pear-shaped and the practice fails to achieve the standards aspired to, that's when the talking starts and pen gets put to paper to prepare an action plan for what happens next year.

It doesn't end there. Just as the PCO inspects the practice, so the nice people at the Commission for Health Audit and Inspection inspect the PCO. The NHS has got more inspectors than Indian Railways!

The point is, the people in the nutcracker are the PCO, so if you work in a practice don't expect too much sympathy if you screw up.

REVIEW AND UPDATE

The quality framework is based on what we know now. In the light of changes to the evidence base, advances in healthcare, changes in legislation or regulation and the need for further clarity, new issues can be included or modifications made. There's going to be one of those independent UK-wide expert groups who will oversee the process. Let's not worry too much about that now!

There's so much more to worry about!

DEVELOPING HUMAN RESOURCES AND MODERNISING INFRASTRUCTURE

DEVELOPING HUMAN RESOURCES AND MODERNISING INFRASTRUCTURE

DOESN'T SOUND MUCH WHEN YOU SAY IT QUICK!

The docs can't do their bit without a lot of other people doing theirs. That is recognised in the contract. There's a touchy-feely bit to make us all believe our working lives will improve and some family-friendly type stuff. Here's what it says:

- helping implement good human resource management practice to improve the working lives of GPs and practice staff, and encourage recruitment and retention
- supporting practices in rural and remote areas
- investment in information management and technology
- better mechanisms to modernise premises.

Where have we heard all that before? Where's the beef? You may well ask. They say the contract will:

- facilitate the introduction of a new career structure
- support the introduction of protected time for skills development
- enable the widespread employment of salaried GPs in GMS where this best suits practice and practitioner preferences

- deliver family-friendly improvements
- encourage recruitment and retention through national schemes such as golden hello schemes, sabbatical schemes, flexible career schemes and returners schemes
- support the development of practice staff including nurses and managers.

☺ *Doing something to support practice staff is welcome and not before time.* In the good old days, when Dr Finlay had his black bag and a drop of Scotch in his tea before doing his rounds, the role of practice staff was very different. Today, it has gone through a huge renaissance. From meeters and greeters to receptionists and typists, practice staff now play a full managerial role in primary care. A fact underlined in the contract.

So much of the practice income will depend on performance of the practice as a whole. Now everyone is in the spotlight, not just the GPs and the nurses. Good news for practice managers.

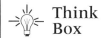 **Think Box**

If you are a GP you will have spent about one fifth of your life being educated and trained to be a GP. What's it like when you first start? They tell me it's exhilarating and fulfilling. However, after you've diagnosed a chesty cough the umpteen thousandth time, you stop feeling like Albert Schweitzer and start getting a bit bored. Is it any wonder these bright darlings get jaded and want to go and do something else?

They're a funny lot, the GPs. They get into being a GP because that's what they want to do. Then they start getting grumpy because there is no career pathway for them. I thought being a GP was a career? I thought being a GP was a specialism. But now we have specialist GPs who go off and do things that GPs don't normally do. Wacky world, or is it me?

The new contract will enable skills development, special interest development *(currently special interest work is done as an add-on, but it looks like it could be made more integral)* and clinical leadership.

Returners will be able to refresh their skills and the gung-ho will be able to slash and crash their way into all sorts of things! What fun! What happened to the chesty cough?

And while the GP is away doing all this good stuff, there is some cash built into the global sum to enable practices to replace the missing doc with another doc. I thought there was a shortage of docs?

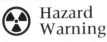 Hazard
Warning

So, sorry Mrs Bloggs, your GP is away having lots of fun on a leadership course. So you'll have to make do with someone else. *(Last warning, stop being cynical – Ed.)*

IT LOOKS LIKE WE CAN ALL LEARN SOMETHING NEW!

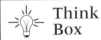 Think
Box

Everyone is going to have protected learning time to extend their roles and facilitate skill mix – paid for out of the global sum. So make sure you get it! Ask how much, when you can go on a course and can you have the entitlement added into your contract of employment.

What's your topic? They will pay for stuff like child protection or cardiopulmonary resuscitation training. Sorry, no basket weaving or fine wine appreciation. Although a foreign language in an ethnic area might be a goer. Give it a try and let me know how you get on!

Practice staff, including nurses, can be trained, groomed, developed and sent home so changed that their other half won't recognise them. Good job too!

Fit as a flea and not ready to give up work? You're in luck. The service is so short of GPs that the fixed retirement age of 70 will be abolished.

You'll be appraised to make sure you're not ga-ga, can tie your shoelaces and know the name of the prime minister.

You can keep going for as long as you are revalidated and can oil your own bandy-chair!

In another attempt to make GP-land more attractive, the global sum will give practices new flexibility to appoint salaried staff.

PCOs can also hire salaried GPs to help them sort out the bits and pieces the other GPs don't want to do.

IMPROVING WORKING LIVES

Great phrase isn't it. Stopping work would improve most people's working life! However, the idea here is to keep everyone working.

Here are the natty wheezes they are going to seduce GPs and their staff with:

- access to NHS childcare
- maternity, paternity, adoptive and special leave
- sick leave arrangements will be reviewed.

. . . There, I bet you feel better already! Quite where all this childcare is going to come from is an interesting question. There is already a national shortage of nursery places. But stand back and watch the new contract negotiators dump another underpants-over-the-trousers job on the luckless souls working in the PCOs – because all this is down to them.

SENIORITY PAYMENTS

The existing seniority payment scheme will be improved to reward experience. The new scheme will deliver a 30% increase in total resources over current spend by 2005/06. The scheme will be based on years of NHS reckonable service. As with the current scheme, the new scheme will recognise the working commitment of general practitioners, with superannuable income being used as a measure of that working commitment. Under these arrangements, GPs who are receiving at least two-thirds of average superannuable income will be entitled to full seniority payments. GPs receiving between one-third and two-thirds of average superannuable income will be entitled to 60% of full seniority payments. GPs in receipt of less than one-third of average superannuable income will not be eligible for the payment.

☺ The existing payment steps will be subject to some *smoothing*. Great word, eh? Not mine, it's out of the BMA's documentation.

WHERE ARE ALL THE GPs GOING TO COME FROM?

There are going to be *golden hellos* (sounds like a mouthwash). They've got to be in place by April 2004. More things for the PCOs to worry about, unless you are in Northern Ireland where they are already in place.

WHAT ABOUT THE WORKERS?

SUPPORTING PRACTICE STAFF: SOME GOOD NEWS!

 Bedtime reading: organisational standards in the quality framework will reward practices for ensuring employment standards comply with good human resources practice in line with *Agenda for Change* principles that are expected to apply to non-medical staff and to prevent exploitation.

In plain English: because there is such a shortage of GPs, nurses are going to be able to do more of what the GPs used to do. I'm not quite clear who is going to do what the nurses used to do – there's a shortage of them too!

Guess what? The good old endless, bottomless pit of money called the global sum will pay to enable practices to develop greater skill mix, with more registered nurses, pharmacists and allied health professionals.

SUPPORTING PRACTICE MANAGERS

At last! I bet you thought you'd been forgotten. No! In this pick 'n' mix world of the new contract, everyone gets a sweetie. Or is it a sweetener . . .?

 If you are a practice manager, make a coffee and read this. It's important. It's the first time you've been recognised!

> 'The new contract will encourage an expanded role for practice management in primary care, supported by the development of practice management competencies. Following consultation with a number of representative organisations a competency framework for practice management has been developed. This competency framework covers strategic issues, the development and delivery of services to patients and practice infrastructure.'

Ooooh, not your cup of tea? Don't panic. It is not envisaged that every practice manager will have, or want, all the competencies. There's a lot of them, and the level of competency increases through the headings: administrative, managerial and strategic.

Here's a summary of what it looks like:

Administrative role	Managerial role	Strategic role
PCT meetings		
Will participate in meetings and possibly take responsibility for implementing action agreed		
	Will coordinate meeting programme, may chair, and will undertake, active management of meeting programme and sub-groups	
		Adopts a strategic approach, convening meetings and reviewing effectiveness and structure. May adopt advisory role
Development plans/reports		
Will provide data for planning/reporting and possibly assist in report production		
	Coordinates production and reviews consistency with external targets/strategy. May initiate remedial action	
		Will participate in policy sub-groups. May take responsibility for co-production and review of contribution to targets
Clinical services		
Will provide data for planning and may assist in service needs assessment		
	Reviews service provision/recommends change. May regularly review and implement developments or service extension	
		Will take responsibility for appropriate service provision and may advise on appropriate provision and development

OK? Got the picture. It's a stepped protocol. There are a host more of them, too many to fill up the book with *(sorry – Ed)*, the full list is on the BMA website. Yup, I know, but it's a web-world these days.

Just to whet your appetite, here are the headings.

> ✓ See, it's a nice long list!
> Well worth taking a look at the detail. Eighty-one sections to keep you entertained and all learned-up!

1 Care pathways
2 Liaison with secondary/tertiary care providers
3 Strategy formulation

4 Innovation
5 Clinical audit
6 Organisational audit
7 Clinical effectiveness (CE)/evidence-based practice (EBP)
8 Resource allocation
9 Professional development
10 Research
11 Health and safety
12 Fire safety
13 Risk assessment
14 Significant event audit/reporting
15 Infection control
16 Confidentiality
17 Ethics
18 Occupational health
19 Poor performance
20 Disaster planning
21 GP time management
22 Locums
23 Partnership meetings
24 Partnership agreement
25 Partnership changes
26 Taxation
27 CPD requirements
28 Reception
29 Information
30 Clinics/health promotion
31 Complaints
32 Community liaison
33 Patient protection
34 Community nursing
35 Social services
36 Working partnership
37 Networking with colleagues from other practices
38 Petty cash
39 Payroll and pensions
40 Invoice payment
41 Insurance
42 Monthly accounting
43 Annual accounts claims/targets/quality payments

44 Drawings
45 Quarterly statements
46 Bank and accountant
47 Cash flow/budgets
48 Staff funding
49 Planning
50 Information
51 Service budgets
52 Deficiency register
53 Resource negotiation
54 Staff management
55 Staff meetings
56 Rotas and work
57 Recruitment and selection
58 Induction and training

. . . and

59 Employment practice
60 Disciplinary and grievance
61 Performance review
62 Pastoral care
63 Supplies
64 Equipment
65 Facilities management and maintenance
66 Facilities provision
67 Security
68 Project management equipment/premises
69 Patient records
70 Data management
71 Data security
72 Data interpretation/manipulation
73 Hardware maintenance
74 GP links
75 Crisis management
76 Project management
77 Health needs assessment
78 Service performance indicators
79 Strategic delivery planning
80 Service prioritisation
81 Resource negotiation

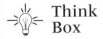 **Think Box**

Let's think about this seriously for a moment.

There are a bewildering range of competencies, but it does mean there should be something there to interest even the least interested.

This is the first time that practice management competencies and development have been recognised in this way. So take advantage of it! It is an opportunity to expand your knowledge. Learn, do stuff and get on. With all this behind you, who knows, one day you might even get a proper job!

 So take some time and think about how you want to develop, what interests you and what you want to do next.

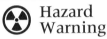 **Hazard Warning**

This type of initiative can look good on paper, send all the right signals and disappear in the dust on someone's shelf. Don't let that happen. Spend time with colleagues and talk with them, get their opinions and make it happen for you all.

Practices will receive funding for practice management through – guess what? Yes:

The global sum!

You can pool resources with other practices and share a practice manager or request access to practice management expertise through the PCO *(another job they can do without)*. There will have to be some new laws to enable some of this. But there shouldn't be a problem, it's technical and not worth worrying about right now.

And if you are working in some country idyll, miles from anywhere, you've not been forgotten in the BMA's cornucopia of new contract good stuff.

The funding formula includes a specific adjustment for rurality. *(Rurality – whose dictionary does that come out of? Rurality!)* This takes account of population sparsity *(that's another dodgy word, isn't it?)* and dispersion.

In England, the development of practice nursing is supported through the document *PCTs Liberating the Talents: helping PCTs and nurses to deliver the NHS*

Plan. Rural and remote GPs will benefit in their global sum and the practice weighted population adjustment to quality payments.

The extra burdens of being a remote and rural GP – for example, extra travel costs to attend PCO-sponsored or PCO-approved training and the continued need to provide out-of-hours care – will be supported by the Out-of-Hours Development Fund.

> ✓ There will be a range of independent contractor and employed options, which will improve upon and replace the current inducement scheme, which will cease on 31 March 2004.

Rural and remote GPs are often more involved in the provision of emergency care outside the setting of their surgery or a local community hospital. This work requires extra training (e.g. BASICS), equipment, resources, commitment and reward. Under the new contract, these services will be commissioned and funded as an enhanced service.

For GPs working for community hospitals and minor injury clinics . . . Staffing of community hospitals and minor injury services is an integral part of many GP practices, particularly in rural or remote areas. Under the new contract these services will be commissioned and funded from the unified budget *or its equivalent in Northern Ireland.*

It's not just the docs in the sticks who have the problems. They have them in the towns, too!

SUPPORTING PRACTICES IN DEPRIVED AREAS

In the now infamous Carr-Hill formula there is a recognition of increased morbidity factors and consequent impact on workload involved in the deprived inner city areas.

MODERNISING INFORMATION MANAGEMENT AND TECHNOLOGY IN GENERAL PRACTICE

OK, LISTEN UP, THIS COULD GET TRICKY

Historically, cash for IT stuff has gone to the practice and GPs with a bit of an interest in computing have spent money on all sorts of kit, some of it very clever and, frankly, some of it rubbish. There are a host of systems out there that can't speak to each other, can't speak to the local hospital and some that can't speak to someone in the next office.

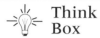

Think Box

Did you know that the NHS IT Tsar, Richard Granger, is the same man who delivered the technology to make the London Congestion Charge work? It was a hugely complicated and controversial project that he delivered on time and in budget. So don't mess with him!

It's going to change. In a nutshell, funding will go to the PCO who, in turn, will be performance-managed by the StHA to make sure the NHS IT Tsar gets his way, hits his time lines and gets the job done.

IT in the NHS is not a hobby any more. About time too! IT is seen as essential to the NHS modernisation agenda.

Think Box

Think about it. If patient notes do become an electronic patient history, warehoused in cyberspace and accessed on a password basis, it means that any authorised person can see a patient's notes. Now, the new contract has already broken the link between the patient and the doctor. Under the new arrangements the patient registers with the practice, not the doctor. If notes can be accessed anywhere, it means patients can be treated anywhere, and the link between the patient and the practice is broken. Then a revolution in healthcare, with doctors competing for patients, becomes a reality.

The gossip is that this was the only part of the new contract that wasn't up for negotiation. The consequences are going to be interesting. There will be a substantial number of GPs and practices who will want to hang on to their systems and probably a battle over access to patient notes.

There will be nationally agreed security and confidentiality conditions which take into account the requirement that information must be available for other medical practitioners looking after patients, subject normally to the patient's informed consent.

Think Box

Informed consent? Funny use of the English language – in the NHS we do it all the time and it is meaningless. How can you have uninformed consent? I think what they mean is 'valid' consent. Sorry to be such a pedant! *(Groan – Ed.)*

Suppliers of NHS IT products will have to pull their socks up. A lot of kit is not interconnective. That means it has no capacity to talk to other kit, which is an essential part of the new NHS IT framework. I can see a lot of bits and pieces ending up in a skip!

It's all very well the PCOs having the money and owning the kit, but with it comes yet another job: they are responsible for the full supporting service, including maintenance, future upgrades, paying for running costs of the new integrated systems and training.

Whilst some GPs are in love with their computer systems, overall it looks to me like the docs have walked away from a load of grief. Nice one!

All this means PCOs will have to come up with:

- service level agreements
- supplier management mechanisms
- nationally accredited systems
- data confidentiality and security
- liability.

Think Box

Who's going to do it? Does the PCO have the expertise? There is a shortage of good IT people in the NHS. A top notch IT wizard in the private sector can earn the kind of money that is enough to run a small country. The NHS pays . . . Well, you know. So get sorted – who is going to do this, do you need to recruit, is there enough work for a full-time post or could you work with another PCO? Or, contract out?

All new systems will be accredited against national standards. Each practice will have guaranteed choice from a number of accredited systems that deliver the required functionality. Such choices will be consistent with local development plans.

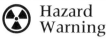 Hazard
Warning

Security is a key issue. The wider use of information held in current practice systems means the development of standards and protocols relating to the access and management of electronic patient records, including the transition from existing arrangements. More work for the PCO and practice managers!

SO, WE'VE GOT ALL THIS NEW KIT, CAN WE USE IT?

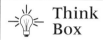 Think
Box

Do you think PCOs are starting to look like Health Authorities?

The initial and continuing education, training and support in the use of IM&T will be managed and funded by – guess who? Our old friends at the PCO! Who else?

The official blurb says 'Mechanisms will be put in place to ensure practice staff are fully supported with continuing training and education'. Well, that's all very good but it seems to ignore the fact that most practice staff have more computing power in their kids' bedrooms than they do on their office desk. And they are very used to buying, banking and browsing on-line. Just because staff can't do IT at work, it doesn't mean they don't do it at home!

Anyway, the training package will ensure staff can:

- use and manage their particular clinical and administrative information systems, including data entry and retrieval
- understand clinical nomenclatures and classifications
- ensure data quality
- implement change management and strategies to enable the move from paper to electronic records
- manage the risks associated with an IT-dependent working environment, including disaster recovery and ensuring operational continuity
- develop and implement workforce strategies to cope with the sum-marisation tasks associated with all clinical data flows into the practice.

If it sounds a bit patronising just think of it as having to fill up the contract with something!

PREMISES

I always think it's strange that the taxpayer funds the GP's place of work, yet ownership remains with the GP and when he sells it the taxpayer never gets a sniff of the capital appreciation. If you thought the new contract would do nothing to change that – you're right!

Indeed, the document says:

> 'Areas with poor returns on capital have historically attracted low levels of investment in primary care infrastructure. To overcome barriers to investment, a first tranche of premises flexibilities has already been introduced. A second tranche was set out in the April 2002 framework. This was designed to overcome hurdles to capital investment in primary care and to enable GPs to move from old to modern premises. These changes have been introduced to maintain GP choice in investment routes and to provide parity in access to funding. It will be implemented from April 2003.'

The flexibilities referred to are:

- the payment of a grant to meet mortgage deficit costs, to enable GPs to sell their existing premises and move to appropriate alternative premises *(that's 'sorting out negative equity' to you and me)*
- the payment of a grant to meet mortgage redemption costs *(this is where the mortgage company may charge a penalty for early redemption)*
- allowing PCOs to take an option on land
- allowing PCOs to continue cost rent payments to GPs who buy premises from a single-handed/two partner practice
- allowing PCOs to review cost rent payments when GPs re-mortgage to lower interest rates
- reimbursement of legal and other professional fees for GPs in new premises developed by public–private partnership
- revised arrangements to pay notional rent in addition to cost rent when premises are modernised or extended
- abatement of notional rent to pay full notional rent on GP capital invested in premises and abated notional rent for NHS capital equivalent to additional costs for heating, lighting, maintenance, etc
- payment of notional rent to leaseholder GPs who improve their premises

- extension of the timescale to repay improvement grants and PMS equivalents to 10 years for owner-occupiers and for renting GPs to renegotiate the terms of their lease to 15 years
- allowing PCOs to directly reimburse insurance and utility costs, maintenance and service charges, etc
- introducing periodic *(potentially quarterly)* reviews of building cost location factors
- introducing index-linked leases *(such as Retail Price Index-based)* to support capital invested in primary care premises better
- a revised premises schedule and a revised commentary
- issuing a letter on safeguards and security for GPs signing leases with third party developers with the intention that PCOs will be able to have a lease assigned to them temporarily if the departing GP is unable to assign it.

In the words of my old Dad: 'A nice little earner'.

QUALITY STANDARDS

Some GP premises are – what shall we say? Quaint? Interesting? Crap? You name it. There are some new standards on the way.

PCOs will inspect premises to make sure practices and consulting rooms meet the new minimum standards. Why should GPs agree to inspections? Well, because there's a few quid around to help improve them, if they fall short of the minimum standards.

This is what the inspectors with the clipboards will be looking for:

	Yup, got it	What?	You must be joking!	Gone to the DIY shop!
1 Practices should take reasonable steps to comply with the Disability Discrimination Act 1995. This includes providing for all users of the building ease of access to premises and movement within them, adequate sound and visual systems for the hearing and visually impaired, and the removal of barriers to the employment of disabled people.				

	Yup, got it	What?	You must be joking!	Gone to the DIY shop!
2 Adequate facilities should also be provided for the elderly and young children, including nappy-changing and feeding facilities.				
3 A properly equipped treatment room.				
4 Properly equipped consulting room for use by the practitioners with adequate arrangements to ensure the privacy of consultations and the right of patients to personal privacy when dressing or undressing, either in a separate examination room or in a screened-off area around an examination couch within the treatment room or the consulting room.				
5 An additional treatment room where enhanced minor injury services are provided.				
6 Practitioners, staff and patients having convenient access, including wheelchair access where reasonably possible, to adequate lavatory and hand washing facilities which meet current infection control standards.				
7 Washbasins connected to running hot and cold water in consulting rooms and treatment areas or in an immediately adjacent room.				
8 Adequate internal waiting areas with enough seating to meet all normal requirements, and provision, either in the reception area or elsewhere, for patients to communicate confidentially with reception staff, including by telephone.				
9 The premises, fittings and furniture to be kept clean and in good repair, with adequate standards of lighting, heating and ventilation.				
10 Adequate arrangements for the storage and disposal of clinical waste.				

	Yup, got it	What?	You must be joking!	Gone to the DIY shop!
11 Adequate fire precautions, including provision for safe exit from the premises, designed in accordance with the Building Regulations agreed with the local fire authority.				
12 Adequate security for drugs, records, prescription pads and pads of doctors' statements.				
13 Where the premises are used for minor surgery or the treatment of minor injuries, a room suitably equipped for the procedures to be carried out.				

 Take a break – make a plan, go on holiday, find another job, buy shares in a building company!

BRANCH OR SPLIT-SITE SURGERIES?

Branch surgeries and outlying facilities can vary in size and quality, and existing or proposed new facilities can improve patient access to services where convenient access to main surgery facilities is difficult.

For a branch surgery to qualify as a second main/split site it must meet the following criteria:

- be open for at least 20 hours a week for provision of medical services automatically entitling it to proper IT support
- meet the minimum standards in the list above
- deliver essential and additional services.

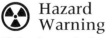 **Hazard Warning**
If the branch doesn't meet the criteria – you've got a problem, as they will not automatically be considered eligible for the funding as a second main/ split-site surgery.

This premises business can go very pear-shaped if the minimum standards aren't met.

It all gets a bit complex. Following public consultation, the premises can be closed.

- A branch surgery can be closed subject to agreement between the PCO and providing practice.
- In the event that there is no agreement the practice can give notice that it wishes to close a branch surgery.
- There will be a given period during which the PCO can issue a counter-notice, to allow for any required consultation, requiring the surgery to remain open until the issue is resolved.

Normal appeal procedures will apply. If the branch surgery is unable to close because a counter-notice was successful, or where both the practice and the PCO agree that the surgery should remain open, then the PCO is required to continue supporting it with the necessary funding.

Branch surgery standards need not be fully met where a practice provides outlying consultation facilities using premises usually used for other purposes.

AND THE PCOS HAVE SOME TEETH

If a PCO carries out an inspection and doesn't like what it sees, it will determine *whether premises accepted for the delivery of services are continuing to meet the relevant standards*. If there are shortcomings:

> 'The LMCs (or GP subcommittee of the Area Medical Committee) will be consulted.'

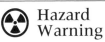 **Hazard Warning**

In short – under most circumstances you've got six months to get your act together. Plenty of time! Noah only needed 30 days to build an ark! In fact, depending on what's wrong, six months is not a long time. You may have to get estimates, the builders in and work out-of-hours. This may not be easy. Negotiate more time if you are likely to need it. Think this through.

Where the shortcomings can be rectified, the practice will agree with the PCO within a month how the shortcomings can be rectified within a reasonable period of time, ensuring that patient safety is not at risk.

If the shortcomings have not been put right within six months (or such longer period as may be agreed between the practice and the PCO), premises payments will cease or be abated, until the shortcomings have been put right.

Oh and, surprise, surprise, there is an appeals procedure . . . I must say the GPs have done a very good deal! Why am I surprised?

INVESTING IN PRIMARY CARE SERVICES

INVESTING IN PRIMARY CARE SERVICES

THERE'S A LOT OF IT ABOUT!

Yes, there's a lot of it about – money, that is. Unprecedented levels of investment are going into the NHS. The first tranche of new money seems to have been eaten up with wage cost inflation. But the Government are determined to see their investment underpinning modernisation of the service. This is very clear in the contract. Money for modernisation that works.

There is a guaranteed UK-wide investment to primary care over a three year period, raising total spend by 33% from £6.1bn to £8.0bn. Three year funding cycles have been a feature of the Chancellor's strategy. Three years gives a longer planning cycle and is a long overdue advance in public sector funding.

The distribution mechanism for primary care is the Carr-Hill resource allocation formula. The foul-ups in the formula, the calculations that showed half of GPs could be worse off, all combined to reduce the negotiations for the contract to near-farce. A lot of egg was left on a lot of faces and the BMA negotiators came in for some stick from their members.

> ☺ Needless to say, the formula is now being tweaked, bench-tested and road-run to a standstill. Men in shaded rooms with wet towels around their heads are working night and day!

The basis of the formula is to recognise the practice workload in the context of the type of patients the practice cares for. This involves complex calculations based on demographics and other arcane sciences.

ADDITIONAL INVESTMENT

UK expenditure on primary care will rise from around £6.1bn in 2002/03 to £8.0bn in 2005/06, and about two-thirds of the increased investment will be spent on rewards for higher quality. This expenditure covers all practices, including PMS practices.

Under the old contract, the Doctors' and Dentists' Review Body (DDRB) made recommendations about changes to the GMS fee scale needed to deliver an Intended Average Net Income (IANI) for GPs, based on the expected level of expenses incurred by GPs.

As you might imagine, this ended up in an almighty mess. Overestimation of GP expenses and other factors have led to overpayment of GPs. According to the DDRB's 2001 report the debt amounted to £7214 per GP. However, the latest Technical Steering Committee (TSC) work shows this figure is now £6688 per GP. Pick a number! Accounting at its finest, don't you think? It's only public money – who cares? *(Me! Ed.)*

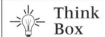 **Think Box**

This nice few quid would have been progressively clawed back under the old contract. The transition from the old contract to the new will see the debt written off. See what I mean!

Wouldn't you have voted for a contract that put six and a half grand in your back-pocket?

ENTER THE GROSS INVESTMENT GUARANTEE

The new contract is based on new investment and the Gross Investment Guarantee ensures that the resources are delivered. Investment in enhanced services will be performance-managed by Strategic Health Authorities (or their equivalents) to ensure *effective and appropriate* deployment.

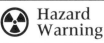 **Hazard Warning**

And if the PCOs don't pull their finger out and develop plans for enhanced services in primary care, the Strategic Health Authority comes in with its size twelve boots and intervenes to ensure that the guaranteed floor is not breached and is spent for the purposes intended.

The purpose of the guaranteed expenditure floor is to develop new services and reward innovation. Any spend on enhanced services where these are currently being funded from GMS monies (excluding LDS) will not count towards the Gross Investment Guarantee.

PCOs will be required to consult their constituent local practices, LMCs and Patient Forums about the level of investment they propose to make on enhanced services and how it will be used in line with the PCO's strategic objectives.

GMS ALLOCATION FORMULA AND THE CARR-HILL FORMULA (AT LAST!)

 This gets labyrinthine! Make a coffee . . .

Let's start with the way it works now. Under the existing contract, practices receive 'per doctor' payments such as the basic practice allowance, capitation fees and item of service payments.

This sounds very sensible, but it does nothing to recognise case mix and differing practice circumstances. Resources follow the distribution of doctors rather than patients and their needs, resources are lost if the number of doctors in a practice reduces, practices do not have security of income (*what self-employed businessman does?*), changes in skill mix are not encouraged and practices have insufficient financial incentives to provide high quality care.

Enter the great hope of the profession. Yes, it's the:

Global Sum!

The global sum payment, combined with new rewards for quality, will address these flaws with a new GMS resource allocation formula, 'Carr-Hill'.

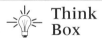 **Think Box**

In case you were wondering, Carr-Hill isn't two people, it's one. It is Professor Roy Carr-Hill of York University. Poor bloke, he's taken such stick over this! His name will live for ever in the history of the NHS. Children will sit on Granddad's knee and ask: 'Where were you when war broke out over the Carr-Hill formula?' The wicked have deliberately confused his name with Benny Hill and there has been endless grief over the calculations. The truth is, it is probably a very good idea!

The Carr-Hill formula takes account of six key factors:

1   patient gender and age for frequency and length of surgery and home
    visit contacts
2   patient gender and age for
    nursing and residential home
    consultations
3   morbidity and mortality
4   newly registered patients
5   unavoidable costs of rurality
6   unavoidable higher costs of
    living through a market forces
    factor applied to all practice staff.

Think Box

Did you know that, on average, newly registered patients generate 40% more workload in the first year? Well, you do now. A factoid to impress everyone with!

To calculate practice entitlement under the global sum, the list size will be multiplied by the practice weighting.

☺ List inflation?
The allocation formula for the global sum will be applied to registered populations from 1 April 2004. The original proposal was that census population information would be used to calculate practices' patient lists, with a commitment to move to registered lists later after allowing time for practices to ensure their lists were accurate. Practices with accurate patient lists felt they were being unfairly penalised by this as there was a deduction across the UK of 6% from all practices for 'list inflation'. Using registered lists is seen by GPs as the fairer method. Meanwhile, it is essential that practices' lists are cleaned so that they are as accurate as possible by April 2004.

Each PCO population will be scaled back to its own census population estimate. PCOs will then scale back the practice lists, taking into account the PCO average list inflation, rather than the national average.

Temporary residents and the provision of immediately necessary and emergency treatment are allowed for in the global sum.

Further unavoidable costs may arise in certain geographical areas, where the physical location of the practice or distance from other healthcare providers means that the practice provides a wider range of services. These will be addressed through additional support for the most isolated and remote practices. Here's what the BMA say about the formula:

'Although we believe the formula to be robust, given the available data, it will inevitably not be a perfect model of the future workload and of the costs that practices may face. When dealing with practice size populations it is very unlikely that any formula could wholly accurately predict demand, due to random fluctuations.'

Does that mean they don't think it works? Dunno, what do you think? They say the formula will be revised in the light of more timely and accurate data being available.

 Hazard Warning

Beyond 2005/06, the additional needs adjustment will take account of new practice-level information on disease prevalence following collection of data in the quality framework.

So make triple sure that you ensure accurate reporting of prevalence in disease registers as this will affect future entitlement under the global sum and quality payments.

IN THE MEAN TIME . . . ENTER THE MINIMUM PRACTICE INCOME GUARANTEE

So, the Carr-Hill formula needs a bit of fine tuning, tweaking, sorting out, modification, alteration, change, adaptation, amendment and hitting with a spanner. In the meantime what happens?

In order to ensure that GPs don't lose any cash and go broke, a minimum guarantee has been inserted – MPIG. Does the MPIG address the anomalies in the formula?

Dr Rob Barnett, Secretary of Liverpool LMC, wrote in *Pulse* magazine in April 2003 about an obvious flaw:

'A practice with an actual list of 4000 and another with a list of 7000 could end up receiving the same value for quality points as if they had a weighted list of 5000.'

MPIG is designed to make sure that no practice loses out financially. However, that is not the point of the new contract. I thought the aim was to make it possible for practices to do better and do more and get paid for it.

Dr Rob underlined the confusion about the role of MPIG. He pointed out that the Red Book payments were translated into the global amount that was used to determine the value of MPIG. However, factors such as appraisal are not costed in the Red Book. There are others – part of the cytology payment and some of the payments for minor operations.

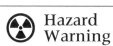 **Hazard Warning**

MPIG will be top sliced by 100 quality points in the year 2004/05 and 150 points the following year. Does this mean that MPIG can really claim to be a minimum income guarantee?

Dr Rob said:

> 'Not all of the payments for practice staff will translate over in the MPIG if a practice undertakes enhanced services or receives high levels of quality payments.'

☺ The good news is, they listened to Dr Rob and quality points have been delinked from the Carr-Hill formula.

Inner-city practices and those with a high proportion of students may find that the Carr-Hill formula works against them. In London, where these issues are common, an additional £18 million is being top sliced but no similar adjustments are being made for other inner-city areas.

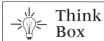 **Think Box**

Well, what do you think?

And now, for the unreconstructed anoraks amongst you, here it is; the Carr-Hill resource allocation formula – go on read it, I dare you!

1   The Carr-Hill formula is founded on an analysis that was used to derive the resource allocations formula for the new GMS contract. It is used to allocate the **global sum** and related payments on the basis of the practice population, weighted for factors that influence relative needs and costs.
    The formula includes the following components:
    • an adjustment for the age and sex structure of the population, including patients in nursing and residential homes
    • an adjustment for the additional needs of the population, relating to morbidity and mortality
    • an adjustment for list turnover
    • adjustments for the unavoidable costs of delivering services to the population, including a staff Market Forces Factor and rurality.
2   The formula differs from those previously developed for resource alloca-tion purposes in two key respects. First, the majority of the formula is to be applied to the four countries within the United Kingdom. Secondly, the formula will be applied to practice populations, rather than Primary Care Organisation populations.
3   The approach to the formula follows that established elsewhere in the field of resource allocation: namely, expressing relative need in cost terms. This involves establishing an age-sex cost curve, estimating the additional resource implications of additional needs, and then adjusting for other factors that affect the cost of delivering services. Given the difficulties of collecting data in this area, a large number of different exercises have been carried out.

Here is a summary of how all this magic was done.

AGE-SEX WORKLOAD CURVE

4   The basis of any allocation formula for a set of services is the population served. For General Medical Services in the UK this is defined by those registered on the lists of each general practitioner. Whilst those lists are well-defined (although there are well-known problems over list inflation) there is no routine dataset that provides the basis for showing the entire workload generated by different age-sex groups on the practice list.
5   Consultations can take place in the surgery, in the patient's own home or in a nursing or residential care home. There is no single data source adequately covering general practice consultations in all of these environ-ments. Whilst there are routine data available on consultations in the surgery, there are only limited data on home visits and no systematic data on nursing and residential home consultations. Consequently they have to be estimated separately, with separate databases.

CONSULTATIONS IN THE SURGERY: ANALYSIS OF THE GENERAL PRACTICE RESEARCH DATABASE (GPRD)

6 The analyses of surgery consultations have been based on the General Practice Research Database (GPRD). It includes data from 240 practices, including eight from Northern Ireland, ten from Wales and twelve from Scotland. The GPRD has individual level consultation frequencies and information on duration has been recorded for all members of the primary care health team in most of the practices since 1999.

7 The whole dataset covers a period from 1996 to August 2002 and contains details of 99 million consultations. However, prior to 1999 the vast majority of the computer systems in these 240 practices did not record when patient files were opened and closed. Of the whole dataset, 69% (68 million) of consultations were time-stamped.

8 It is important to emphasise that the GPRD material refers to 'consultations', but these are simply instances of a patient's computer file being accessed. So a receptionist checking an appointment or a computer manager doing data checks will both count as 'consultations'. They are more properly referred to as 'file openings'.

9 It can be argued that the relative GP workload associated with different patient groups may be approximated by the times for which the files were open and that these data may also be used to estimate consultation rates. The obvious objections are that the opening of a patient's computer file may not denote a consultation and that the length of time for which the file is opened may not reflect the workload associated with the event being recorded.

An example of the latter would be the retrospective entering of details of a home visit. The retrospective entering of home visit details is unlikely to reflect the full workload of home visits, which are often longer than surgery visits and also have an associated travel time. For this reason, home visits have been treated separately.

The age-sex workload adjustment is in the table below.

Table 1: Mean total time for which a patient file was opened in minutes per year: all staff, weighted by staff input cost

	Males – Average time per person	Ratio to male 5–14	Females – Average time per person	Ratio to male 5–14
0–4	50.38	3.97	46.31	3.65
5–14	12.69	1.00	13.35	1.05
15–44	14.64	1.15	31.00	2.44
45–64	30.65	2.42	48.28	3.80
65–74	53.81	4.24	62.38	4.92
75–84	58.62	4.62	63.06	4.97
85+	29.16	2.30	29.14	2.30

10   The counter-intuitive reduction in average time (and hence relative
      workload) for the most elderly patients could be explained by a higher
      proportion of very short file openings for those groups to record other
      information about the patient. Furthermore, these may refer to home or
      care home visits, the details of which are recorded *post hoc* and do not
      reflect the actual workload generated by home visits.

HOME VISITS

11   As discussed above, the GPRD does not adequately record home visits.
      Although the file may be opened in relation to home visits, this is likely to
      be for a relatively short period, as the information is added after the home
      visit has taken place. This will therefore not reflect the full workload
      impact of the home visit.

LENGTH OF THE HOME VISIT

12   On the whole, a home visit tends to generate a higher workload than a
      surgery consultation, as the consultation itself is often longer and a home
      visit also has an associated travel time. According to the 1992/93 GP
      workload survey, the average length of a home visit, including travel time,
      is 25.2 minutes.

VARIATION BY AGE AND SEX

13   The most extensive data available on home visits are those from
      Morbidity Statistics for General Practice 4 (1991/92). A clear 'J'-shaped
      relationship between age and home visiting rates is apparent for both males
      and females.

Table 2: Home visit rates per 1000 patient years

	0–4	5–15	16–24	25–44	45–64	65–74	75–84	85+
Male	498	126	56	63	136	506	1331	2792
Female	454	128	150	163	200	608	1628	3081

14   Applying the home visit length to these weights and combining with the
      consultations in surgery produces an age-sex workload index, which is set
      out in Table 3. The formula uses different age-sex workload indices in
      Scotland and these are shown in Table 4.

Table 3: Age-sex Workload Index (males aged 5–14 = 1): UK less Scotland

	0–4	5–14	15–44	45–64	65–74	75–84	85+
Male	3.97	1.00	1.02	2.15	4.19	5.18	6.27
Female	3.64	1.04	2.19	3.36	4.90	6.56	6.72

Table 4: Age-sex Workload Index (males aged 5–14 = 1): Scotland

	0–4	5–14	15–24	25–44	45–64	65–74	75–84	85+
Male	2.510	1.000	1.153	1.272	1.823	2.672	3.207	3.468
Female	2.240	1.102	2.371	2.524	2.714	3.067	3.342	3.340

NURSING AND RESIDENTIAL HOMES

15   Two separate surveys were carried out to analyse the relative workload
     generated by patients in nursing and residential homes. One was directed
     to nursing and residential homes, to generate information on the
     frequency of consultations, and the other to GPs, looking at time spent
     in nursing and residential home consultations. Overall, patients in nursing
     and residential homes generate more workload than patients with other-
     wise similar characteristics who are not in nursing and residential homes.
     This is mainly due to the fact that all nursing and residential home
     consultations involve travelling time. The workload factor applied to
     patients in nursing and residential homes is 1.43.

LIST TURNOVER

16   Areas with high list turnover often have higher workload, as patients in
     their first year of registration in a practice tend to have more consultations
     than other patients with otherwise similar characteristics.

17   The impact of list turnover was analysed using the GPRD, which contains
     data on patient registration date. The results of this analysis indicate that
     the average time in 'consultation' is some 40–50% higher for patients in
     their first year of registration in the practice compared with other patients.
     The rate varies across age and sex bands, with young males having the
     strongest additional effect. Rather than create an entirely separate age-sex
     cost curve for new registrations, the average uplift of a factor of 1.46 will
     be applied to all new registrations.

ADDITIONAL NEEDS

18 As well as the impact on practice workload generated by differing age and sex groups, the impact of indicators of mortality and morbidity on consultation frequency has been modelled.

19 This has been modelled using the Health Survey for England data between 1998 and 2000. The survey asks participants whether they have had a GP consultation in the past two weeks, and, if yes, the number of such consultations. The survey also includes information on age, sex, geographic location and a range of socio-economic indicators. These were combined with a range of other small area level explanatory variables, including census variables, mortality rates, and supply variables. The analysis was conducted at ward level, and wards were excluded where there were less than five observations in the ward. This reduces the sample size to 2404 wards.

20 Of the variables tested, Standardised Limited Long-standing Illness (SLLI) and the Standardised Mortality Ratio for those aged under 65 (SMR < 65) were found to be significant and the best at explaining variations in workload over and above age and sex. They are related to workload by the following formula:

Practice list adjusted for list inflation

$$* \; ((48.1198) + (0.26115 * SLLI)$$
$$+ (0.23676 * SMR < 65))$$

scaled back to the UK population.

21 Special provision is being made for Scotland. The evidence shows that although the Standardised Mortality Ratio helps to explain variations in additional need in Scotland, other factors perform better in combination with it than Standardised Limited Long-standing Illness. Thus in Scotland, the explanatory variables used in addition to Standardised Mortality Ratio for those aged under 65 (SMR < 65) are:

• unemployment rate
• elderly people on income support (aged 65 or more)
• households with two or more indicators of deprivation.

UNAVOIDABLE COSTS

22 As well as the impact on workload of practice characteristics, it is also necessary to analyse the impact on costs. Practices are likely to face differing costs of delivering a service depending on location and structure. Within the global sum, we believe there to be three main causes of this: market forces, rurality and practice size.

Staff market forces factor

23   The aim of the staff MFF component is to reflect the geographical variation in staff costs that practices will incur. The Market Forces Factor (MFF) adjustment will be used to compensate for this. The MFF was developed by the University of Warwick, using the same methodology as that used for general NHS allocations.

24   The staff MFF is based on the latest three years of the New Earnings Survey Panel Dataset. The latest three years of data are used and estimates are given in terms of three year averages. The analysis uses individual earnings of full-time employees aged 16–70 in the private sector whose pay is not affected by absence. Regression analysis is then carried out to isolate the impact of geographical area on costs, controlling for the effect of other factors such as age, sex, industry and occupation.

25   The results have then been smoothed to prevent cliff-edge effects between neighbouring areas among the 173 zones used in the analysis. This reflects the fact that the labour market pressures in one area are likely to be influenced by those of its neighbours. This element of the formula has been given a weighting of 48%, as this is the average proportion of the global sum accounted for by practice staff expenses. The adjustment does not apply to general practitioners or non-staff expenses.

26   The equivalent earnings dataset for Northern Ireland was not amenable to similar analysis. The MFF for Northern Ireland outside Belfast has therefore been taken as the average 103 between Scotland and Wales, outside of Edinburgh and Cardiff respectively, whilst the MFF for Belfast has been taken to be the average between Edinburgh and Cardiff.

Rurality

27   The rurality of the practice population is also likely to have an influence on the costs of delivering services. The impact of rurality on costs has been modelled using Inland Revenue information on GP expenses. This is under the assumption that rurality acts as an unavoidable cost, impacting on the expenses associated with delivering services. Because it only applies to the expenses element of GMS expenditure, this adjustment has been given an overall weighting of 58%.

28   The dataset contained information on around 20 000 GPs across England, Scotland and Wales. This was aggregated to practice level using practice identifiers. The impact of population density (persons per hectare in the wards from which a practice draws its patients) and dispersion (average distance of patients to practice, in 100 metre units) indicators was modelled against GP expenses. The modelling controlled for other factors such as the age and deprivation structure of the population, market forces, and other characteristics such as dispensing status and list size. The nature

of the relationship between rurality and expenses is such that the equation explaining it works best when the data are transformed into logarithms. The estimated coefficients on the logarithms of population density and dispersion reflect the 'unavoidable cost' of the rurality and remoteness of the area. Thus, for given population densities and dispersions, variations in the unavoidable costs associated with rurality are explained by the following formula:

Practice list adjusted for list inflation
$* ((0.05 * \log \text{average distance})$
$- (0.06 * \log \text{population density}))$
scaled back to the UK population.

29   For Scotland, the formula includes an additional component relating to economies of scale for a limited number of practices.

OTHER ISSUES

Practice size (economies of scale)

30   Small practices can be expected to incur disproportionately high expenses due to their inability to secure economies of scale. Many costs (particularly those associated with premises) are not easily disaggregated and must be incurred irrespective of practice size. Using data from the Inland Revenue on Schedule D expenses by practice list size, a strong diseconomies effect was detected at low list sizes. This effect would, if imported wholesale into the formula, have had a dramatic and potentially undesirable impact on the distribution of the global sum, notwithstanding that, by definition, it would be applied only to expenses (58% of spend).

The case for including the unavoidable costs associated with diseconomies of scale in the formula was rejected in order to avoid any perverse incentives for practices to disaggregate or to avoid amalgamation.

London

31   Special provision is being made for London. A sum (of about £18 million) has been set aside to recognise the potentially destabilising effects of the implementation of the Carr-Hill formula. This sum will be distributed amongst practices in London on the basis of practice populations after adjustment for list inflation, unweighted for age, sex or additional need.

Combining the adjustments

32   Each adjustment will generate a separate practice index, comparing the practice score on the adjustment to the national average. The indices are then simultaneously applied to the practice list.

33   This will produce the practice weighted population. The application of the
     indices to all practices will produce an overall notional population which
     differs from the actual UK population as estimated by the Office for
     National Statistics (ONS). Weighted populations are adjusted so as to
     total to that ONS population – a process known as normalisation.*

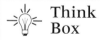 Well? Did you read it? Well done! It is interesting, isn't it, how much
data has come from Inland Revenue records. So, the accuracy of the
formula may depend on GPs' accounts being wholly accurate!

Interesting, too, that the tables for Scotland are only really different
because they divide their age groups up differently to the rest.

This work has come in for some real stick, but for NHS anoraks (like you!)
it is fascinating and the first time there has been an attempt to evolve
formulae in this way. When the NHS gets its IT act together, the whole thing
will become a lot easier.

Now, go and find someone you can dazzle with your knowledge of the
New Earnings Survey Panel Dataset!

GLOBAL SUM PAYMENTS

The global sum includes provision for the delivery of essential and additional
services, staff costs, locum reimbursement including for appraisal, career
development, and protected time. Provision for uplifting non-medical staff
costs as a result of the principles of *Agenda for Change* has been, and will
continue to be, included in the arrangements for revising the global sum.

The funding flow is important to understand. Resources will be allocated
to PCOs who, in turn, *will be obliged* to allocate resources to practices in
accordance with UK-wide arrangements guaranteed in law.

**Think
Box**

An average UK practice, with an average practice weighted population,
will receive £300 000 in 2004/05/06, an average per patient of £50.

Don't forget, there is a balance between the money allocated through the
global sum and the likely potential for achieving higher rewards within the
quality and outcomes framework.

So when you are doing your sums on the back of a fag packet you should
take into account not only the resources you are likely to receive through

---

* As we went to press, normalisation bit the dust, redundant following the move to the use of
  registered lists.

the global sum, but also the substantial potential income from the delivery of quality and the provision of enhanced services.

There is an agreed muddle with the Carr-Hill formula right now but they have to get it right as the formula will be implemented in full from 2004/05!

In the elegant prose of the BMA: 'The formula inevitably has a significant redistributive effect at PCO and practice level, given the shift from largely doctor-based allocations to patient needs-based allocations.'

You can say that again. The new arrangements could destabilise existing practices, particularly in those areas which have been under-resourced under the existing funding arrangements.

FUNDING FLOWS

The pricing of the contract is fixed and not subject to PCO discretion; the entitlements are guaranteed, many enshrined in regulations or legal determinations.

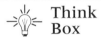

Think Box

If all the practices hit all the maximum quality targets, will there be enough money in the kitty to pay up, or is the Treasury banking on some slow starters and poor performers?

How will it work? A total sum in respect of GMS services will be allocated to each PCO as part of an enlarged unified budget allocation. This allocation method will replace the existing arrangement whereby PCOs draw down money from the Health Departments according to the fees and allowances paid. So those nasty people at the PCO can't hang onto practice cash!

It is the same with quality payments. PCOs will receive full funding from the Health Departments, allocated on the basis of the Carr-Hill formula. They will be responsible for distributing this element of their budget and will be required by law to pay practices the fixed reward per point.

PREMISES

All premises funding will form part of a single fund in each country from 2004/05, *subject to primary legislation*. This fund will operate alongside the global sum and the quality framework. In England, a lead PCT within each Strategic Health Authority will hold the resources for premises on behalf of all PCTs. Decisions on the distribution of these funds to individual PCTs will be subject to joint arrangements with the Strategic Health Authority.

Existing spend and additional funds needed to support new projects that have already been agreed between practices and PCTs will be guaranteed to PCTs as a baseline (being prepared with the Valuation Office Agency).

PENSIONS

Here's a quick teach-in on docs' pensions . . .

GPs' pensions are calculated under a career earnings method rather than a final salary scheme. Each year of pensionable income is increased by an *uprating* or *dynamising* factor on a cumulative basis.

The *uprating* factor is currently based on year-on-year changes in the Intended Average Net Income (IANI). An accrual rate is then applied on retirement age to the individual GP's total *uprated* career earnings to provide an annual pension entitlement.

In addition, a tax-free lump sum of three times the annual pension is payable. Once a pension is being paid, it is uprated annually by retail price inflation.

OK? Got that. Seems like a good deal?

Well, many GPs don't think so. Because:

- the pensions are unfair relative to the pensions that consultants receive, given their respective NHS earnings
- their pensions do not take account of all NHS earnings, unlike the pensions of their PMS counterparts, and some locum work is not super-annuable
- practice manager partners are excluded from the scheme, as are staff who work for not-for-profit GP out-of-hours cooperatives which provide services to the NHS

- the uprating factor is not based on changes year-on-year in all NHS earnings
- differences between how officer and practitioner pensions are calculated can militate against the development of portfolio careers.

So, they're gonna change it. This is the new definition of pensionable pay:

- delivering services as a GMS or PMS provider, excluding work delegated to others
- delivering services under delegation directly from GMS or PMS providers, including locum work
- board, advisory or other work, including delivering services carried out under employment with PCOs or other NHS bodies
- work carried out as NHS services under the collaborative arrangements with Local Authorities
- practice-based work carried out in educating or in organising the education of medical students, undergraduate, vocational and postgraduate training funded through national levies or otherwise.

Regulations will also shortly be changed to enable GP locum earnings to become pensionable retrospectively back to 2002/03.

And for the real brain-boxes this is how superannuable profits are calculated:

> 'GPs will make monthly payments on account to the Pensions Agency for their employer and employee superannuation contributions. When the practice accounts have been finalised, the practice accountants will produce a certificate of NHS profits in specified form to be forwarded to the Pensions Agency with any balance in payment.'

 Think Box

In the current pensions environment it looks to me as if this is a very good deal indeed! A lot of GPs who might have taken early retirement are staying on because the new pension arrangements are so attractive.

In the long run, is funding for such a generous scheme sustainable?

BETTER SERVICES FOR PATIENTS

BETTER SERVICES FOR PATIENTS

Everyone tells me the contract is a great deal for patients. I'm going to take some persuading. Any contract that allows GPs to opt out of what I regard as foundation services, in my view can't be a good deal for patients.

Perhaps I'm wrong? Let's take a look . . .

This is what the BMA says:

> 'The new GMS contract offers many benefits for family doctors and other members of the primary health care team. But its ultimate purpose is to improve patient care.'

Ultimate purpose? Hmmm . . .

The contract calls for:

- the allocation of resources to practices according to patients' needs
- choice of practice supported by better information
- choice of practitioner
- a Patient Services Guarantee, and access to a wider range of services
- higher quality services
- the collection of patients' experience through practice surveys and involvement in service development
- a programme of initiatives involving patients to manage demand for services.

Let's take 'em one at a time.

ALLOCATION OF RESOURCES TO MEET PATIENTS' NEEDS

Under the new contract, resources for the basic practice infrastructure will be allocated to practices on the basis of the weighted needs of their patient population – the famous Carr-Hill formula.

With the exception of premises and IM&T, resources for the infrastructure costs of staffing and basic operating costs will be allocated to practices on the weighted needs of the population they serve.

This will be independent of the number of doctors in the practice. This is important because if a doctor, nurse or staff member leaves the practice, the resources will remain. This gives the practice a chance to reorganise the service. Yup, that's a win for patients. (And for the docs, who can redistribute the cash between them and soldier on!)

The BMA claim the famous global sum funding arrangements will also mean that practices have greater flexibility to organise their services in whatever way best enables them to deliver high quality services for their patients. This is OK provided the patients have a big say in the 'organising'.

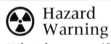 **Hazard Warning**

What happens if all the local practices have closed lists? Patients have to throw themselves on the mercy of the PCO to come up with a solution.

Patients will continue to be free to register with any local practice that is open and practices will continue to have discretion over new patient registrations. No change there, then.

By law PCOs will have to produce information about different practices and the practice will have to produce a practice leaflet.

Think Box

How do you find out about the right doctor for you and your family? A leaflet? No! You ask the other mums at the school gates or talk to folk at the day centre about which practice is good for the elderly. Forget leaflets – they just cost money. Patient aren't stupid; they gossip, network and ask around!

If a practice wants to close a list, the new contract introduces a formal, transparent process to establish list closure. The proposed closure can be reviewed by an assessment panel and there is a specific right of appeal against an adverse assessment to the Strategic Health Authority.

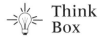

	Think
	Box

Does this help patients? Depends on how long the process takes and the likely attitude of a practice that has tried to close its list and been forced to keep it open.

HOW DO YOU CLOSE A LIST?

STAGE ONE

Within seven days of a notification by a practice that it may wish to close its list, talks begin with the PCO about what additional support the practice could receive to keep its list open and the options for alternative provision. Talks shouldn't go on beyond 28 days.

STAGE TWO

If the practice and PCO agree that list closure is inevitable, the practice submits a closure notice. When such a notice has been served, it cannot be withdrawn within a period of three months unless the PCO agrees.

Within 14 days of receiving the notice, the PCO must either:

- approve the closure notice, in which case the practice list closes either for a period of 12 months, or until the number of patients recorded on the practice list has reduced by a percentage of the practice list size agreed by the PCO and the practice, or until the list size has fallen to the lower limit of an agreed specified range, which will apply for a 12-month period, or by agreement otherwise between the practice and the PCO, or
- reject the closure notice, in which case the notice will be remitted immediately for determination by an assessment panel under the dispute resolution procedures.

STAGE THREE

Where necessary, each PCO will establish an assessment panel, both to consider practice closure notices which have been rejected by the PCO and to determine how requests for new patient registrations should be dealt with where there is mass closure.

What wise heads are needed to accomplish this little task(!)?

- a PCO Chief Executive
- a patient representative (where do they come from – usual suspects or someone off a bus queue?)
- an LMC representative
- a Director from the Strategic Health Authority.

. . . If you are ever on one of these panels, don't forget to visit the practice!

The great and the good have to make their minds up in 28 days.

In the end the panel can either:

- agree that the list may close within seven days, or
- disagree, in which case the list will remain open and offer support to the practice.

Not exactly rocket science, is it? The practice will not normally be able to reapply for list closure within three months from the date of the determination of the panel, unless there is a significant change in circumstances.

Practices with closed lists will have a fast-track right of appeal (within seven days) to the Strategic Health Authority against an adverse decision made by the assessment panel in respect of forced allocations.

Is this any good for patients? Well, it's unsettling at the very least. It is important that patients continue to have access to primary medical services and they will continue to have access to services under the immediate/necessary/emergency rules.

REMOVAL OF PATIENTS

When it all turns nasty, or in the official language, when there is an *irreconcilable breakdown*, the practice can kick the patient out.

Patients have to:

- receive a warning before removal
- be given specific reasons by the practice as to why they've had the order of the boot.

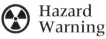 Hazard
Warning

The practice has a right to remove a violent patient. This is extended to safeguard all those who might have reasonable fears for their safety. These will now include members of the practice's staff, other patients and any other bystanders present where the act of violence is committed or the behaviour takes place. Violence includes actual or threatened physical violence or verbal abuse leading to a fear for a person's safety.

And guess who picks up the pieces? The PCO. They have to ensure that there is a service available for patients who are difficult to manage, and this will be commissioned separately as an enhanced service.

CHOICE OF PRACTITIONER

Patients will now register with practices rather than individual GPs. They can only request to be seen by a practitioner of their choice.

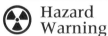 Hazard
Warning

I once saw some very interesting data from the Small Practices Association, that patients do better when they have a good relationship with the doctor. Under the new arrangements, visit your practice seven times and you stand a good chance of seeing seven different doctors.

Patients who exercise their right to see the practitioner of their choice may have to wait longer to see their preferred practitioner. Not so good.

Why make the change? To get more patients through the system. It creates an organisational flexibility.

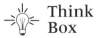 **Think Box**

So far, this all seems to be about getting rid of patients and closing lists. Is that consistent with the BMA's ultimate objective to improve patient care?

What really makes for good patient care? What do you look for in a doctor or practice?

Write down the five most important things and use them as a yardstick to measure where you work, or what you manage:

1
2
3
4
5

THE PATIENT SERVICES GUARANTEE

There's a lot more money going into primary care – how will it translate into better services for the customer? The Patient Services Guarantee is the answer. Is it a guarantee? A promise, a pledge? Can we get our money back if it doesn't work? You must be joking!

Here's the BMA speaking on the topic:

> 'The new GMS contract is a UK-wide contract. The aim is to ensure that patients receive a consistent range of high quality services throughout the UK. The contract does, however, recognise that certain services are provided in different areas in response to local need.
>
> The new contract will ensure that patients have access to a wide range of services delivered in primary care settings. In addition, the quality and outcome rewards in the new contract will incentivise good chronic disease management and holistic personal care within general practices. Patients who need continuity of care will be able to receive it.'

If that doesn't sound too earth-shattering, it's because it isn't! There's a bit more that's interesting – it's all about GP workload. See – it would be lovely if the patients didn't keep getting in the way!

'The mechanisms will enable more flexible configuration of services across PCOs. These are designed to recognise that many practices are facing considerable challenges in managing increasing workload. Combined with the introduction of better human resource management policies, including measures to improve the recruitment and retention of GPs, they will help ensure that primary care capacity is expanded. This will enable better services to be delivered to patients.'

Convinced? No, neither am I. Because this is what they are leading up to:

'It is expected that most practices will deliver the full range of additional services. *However, where practices have no other option, they may opt out of the provision of one or more defined additional services.* In these circumstances, *the PCO is responsible for ensuring that the Patient Services Guarantee is delivered.*'

So, once again, the PCO has to pick up the pieces. Oh, and the guarantee? What does it actually guarantee? Well, er, nothing:

'This guarantee states that "patients will continue to be offered at least the range of services that they currently enjoy under the existing contract."'

So, in other words, all this new money going into primary care, all this upheaval, messing about and sweat, and all the patient receives is a *guarantee* that they will get what they've always got and maybe it will be provided by a complete stranger in another location.

Is it just me, or is the world going mad?

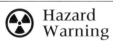 **Hazard**
Warning

The PCOs have got their work cut out here. They will have to be really on top of what practices are and are not going to do. You can bet your last shilling that if the practice ain't gonna do it, there will be a very good reason. That reason will be staff, logistics or money. PCOs will collect a good few headaches trying to conjure up staff, money and locations. Looks to me like a 'bog-standard' healthcare system may not be too far away.

PCO managers are good but they are not magicians.

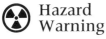 **Hazard**
Warning

It gets worse! The so-called guarantee will be backed up in primary legislation by a new legal duty on PCOs. Get that? A legal duty on the PCO, not the doctor or the practice. It is a legal duty for the PCO!

How the &*%% did that happen?

OH, AND CHOICE?

The great mantra of the modern NHS is choice and it is not missing from the new contract. Call this choice? It's choice about getting treatment from anywhere but the family doctor!

'**Where possible** and **practicable**, patients who require it **will be given choice**, in particular, for single or short duration healthcare episodes and problems. This will be achieved through enabling patients to use alternatives such as NHS walk-in centres, NHS Direct, NHS24 or community pharmacists as complementary alternatives to attending the surgery.'

In other words, clear off someplace else?

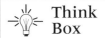 **Think**
Box

How did it come to this? The truth is, as sorry as I am to see the demise of the family doctor, not enough docs want to be family doctors and there are too many patients. The new contract is really a thinly disguised pay rise for docs, including sneaky ways of getting their workload done by other people, in the hope that it will encourage more docs to become, and to stay, a GP.

The risk is that it is very wage cost inflationary and gambles that the PCOs can fill the gaps.

Will it work?

So in answer to the question, is there a guarantee? Well, there is an assurance but no real security, there is law but no contract and there is a realisation that the docs are just not going to keep doing what they used to do and we'd better get used to someone else doing what they once did.

Shame, ain't it?

HIGHER QUALITY SERVICES

Of course, we can't have a health publication without banging on a bit about quality. It is obligatory. So, here it is!

The BMA say:

> '. . . substantial additional investment will support the imple-
> mentation of a wide-ranging quality framework based on latest
> research evidence. This will help ensure excellent management
> of a wide range of chronic diseases. It will have a very significant
> impact in improving clinical outcomes for patients. It will also
> help avoid unnecessary referrals to hospitals.
>
> The organisational standards will also provide assurance to
> patients that practices are well run. The investment in premises
> and the quality standards attached to the new premises flex-
> ibilities will help ensure that patients receive care in a high
> quality physical environment.'

Frankly, if I need a trip to the GP, I can put up with a bit of fluff in the corner and an out-of-date magazine or two. Bunging GPs huge bundles of cash to tart up their consulting rooms is a good move if you are a GP and own the premises. Never mind the carpet, what about the consultation?

And, whilst we are in a quality frame of mind, the Gods of General Practice tell us it is considered good practice to book consultations at 10 minute intervals. Docs are now set to get some cash if they can stick to the 10 minute target.

HOW WAS IT FOR YOU?

 Think Box

I can't see anything on 'Was the doc rude?' or 'Were his hands cold?'!

Finding out what the patient experience is like is not a bad idea and the simplest way of doing it is to ask the punters what they thought. Patients will be asked their opinion of:

- the physical environment
- the convenience and accessibility of the services
- the practice/patient relationship
- the helpfulness of support staff
- the appropriateness and timeliness of the whole episode of care.

☺ PCO managers need to know there are two accredited patient questionnaires that have been tested and approved through a process of peer review. Apparently, they have been shown to have real benefits, not just in creating an opportunity to assess patients' views, but also in alerting the practice to both strengths and weaknesses.

One less job to worry about . . .

WORKING IN PARTNERSHIP

This is one of those good old NHS euphemisms for 'get someone else to do it'.

The docs have woken up to the fact that if they are going to be able to expand primary care, manage their workload and earnings to suit themselves, and improve their availability to patients, something has got to give. This is a circle that no one can square.

What's the answer? Enable patients to manage their own conditions! Yes, I promise I am not making it up. 'Patients can manage their own conditions.' Well, I guess they are the experts?

There's more. There is an understanding that 'not enough GPs' means other people are going to have to do what the docs can't do, or don't want to do. Services could be offered by other health professionals.

The BMA thinks this is a good idea where 'services could be accessed more easily'. And more cost-effectively. So it's about saving money, then?

Well, it's about spending money to save money. They have a special £10m ring-fenced fund looking for examples of good practice, where what the GP did is being done by somebody else.

They are looking for/at:

- development of minor illness management and self-care education programmes by professionals such as nurses, therapists, pharmacists and paramedics
- development and support for Expert Patient initiatives to make better use of primary care and general practice, building on the evaluation and roll-out of the current national scheme, but extending its principles to more local practice-driven schemes

- supporting non-GP based chronic disease management schemes aimed at helping to manage ongoing, and develop new, secondary prevention initiatives
- promoting effective use of health services, better patient communication, and better self-care
- evaluating how patients use services and understanding how best to communicate with them about effective use of, and changes in, services.

☺ . . . and, at last, an attempt to reduce the number of people who get sick in the first place. Included in the list is an 'aim to encouraging a culture shift in public involvement in their own health care management, improving people's ability to use the NHS appropriately and increasing the number of those in future generations who choose careers in the NHS'. The initiative is aimed at providing imaginative and impartial health education and training to teachers, parents and pupils via the National Curriculum.

Which great man said 'all real change starts in the school playground'?

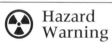 **Hazard Warning**

OK, so you are a brave PCO manager at a public meeting explaining how the new contract will make the patient experience all lovely and gorgeous.

Just how will you get around explaining to a startled audience, whose taxes have gone through the roof to pay for better public services, that the contract is full of ideas for palming patients off someplace else, with a guarantee that doesn't give them any more than they've got now and isn't really a guarantee anyway – and by the way, they'll have to register with an organisation and not a person and some services will be provided in a Portakabin on the other side of town? . . . Good luck!

Please write your answer here, frame it and send it to me!

UNDERPINNING THE CONTRACT — NUTS AND BOLTS

UNDERPINNING THE CONTRACT — NUTS AND BOLTS

UNDERPINNING THE CONTRACT — NUTS AND BOLTS

This is the chapter that the anoraks have been waiting for. It's all the detail stuff and the cogs that make it all work. To ensure that readers do not lose the will to live I have done my best to pare it down to the minimum. It's the sort of Naked Guru bit – with apologies to Jamie Oliver.

 Let's get a cup of coffee on the go and plough through. We will look at:

- the nature and contents of the contract
- who can provide services
- vacancies and practice splits
- contract review arrangements
- how the list arrangements for professionals will be rationalised
- mechanisms for dispute resolution and appeals
- the role of LMCs and Area Medical Committee GP subcommittees
- changes needed to primary legislation.

Get these eight points under your belt, make a set of PowerPoint slides and step forth into the world as the guru's guru and the doyen of the speaking circuit!

NATURE AND CONTENTS OF THE CONTRACT

The current GMS contract is a collection of statutory arrangements made by the Health Departments of the four countries between PCOs and individual GPs. A fundamental change in the new GMS contract is that in future practices will enter into contracts with their local PCO. This requires the existing statutory arrangements to be replaced.

> ☼ ☺ The April 2004 start point does not prevent earlier implementation of many of the proposals. To ease your furrowed brow, there is a timetable at the back of the book (*see* page 133).

Existing GMS practices will transfer to the new contract on 1 April 2004.

The contract and supporting documentation will set out, either directly or by reference to an external source (e.g. the Carr-Hill formula), the agreement between the practice and the PCO. Here's what has to be in it:

- which services will be provided, in the light of the new arrangements around
- service commissioning
- the level of quality of essential and additional services that the practice aspires to deliver
- the support arrangements to be provided, including human resource management, IM&T, premises and support for rural and remote GPs
- the total financial resources that the practice will receive.

> 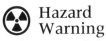 **Hazard Warning**
>
> It is expected that the contract will normally take the form of an NHS contract (in Northern Ireland, a Health and Social Services contract) rather than a private law contract, following granting of Health Service Body status. Where there is an NHS contract, this means practice disputes on contractual matters that are not resolved locally will be resolved through the StHA rather than the courts. It is anticipated that most GMS providers will opt for these contracts but no one will be forced down this route and, *if the practice requires, the new GMS contracts can be ordinary contracts at law.*

The UK contract will permit local variations for the provision of local enhanced services.

☺ One great new idea in the contract *(Just one? Ed)* – practices will be allowed to have other primary care professionals, including nurses and practice managers, sign up as parties to the contract.

The practice-based contract is fundamental to the new arrangements. It will permit the allocation of the global sum monies, and will mean that, should a GP within a practice retire, it will be for the practice to decide how best to continue to meet its service obligations, rather than the PCO advertising and appointing GPs to vacancies, as at present. *Whilst partnership law would allow one partner to sign on behalf of the whole practice, it is envisaged that all partners will have to sign the contract.*

PROVIDERS OF SERVICES

This is really arcane but it's important:

1 a GMS contract is with the provider, made up of one or more individuals who act in their personal capacity
2 a provider must always include at least one general medical practitioner holding a Joint Committee on Postgraduate Training (JCPTGP) certificate (or who is suitably experienced within the meaning of section 31 of the National Health Service Act 1977 (or its equivalent))
3 a provider must be constituted from individuals from within the NHS though not necessarily from a clinical discipline, for example a practice manager.

A provider unit will, subject to point (2) above, be made up of one or more of the following groups:

(a) a general practitioner (defined as a registered medical practitioner on the GP Register, subject to the introduction of proposed legislation, or suitably experienced in the interim) together with one or more persons listed in (b), (c), and/or (d)
(b) a healthcare professional (defined as a person who is a member of a profession regulated by one of the regulatory bodies referred to in section 25(3) of the NHS Reforms and

Health Care Professions Act 2002), who provides services to
the NHS

(c)   an individual employed by an NHS Trust, Foundation Trust
or PCT or equivalent body in Scotland, Wales and Northern
Ireland; a GMS or GDS contractor or equivalent body in
Scotland, Wales and Northern Ireland; a PMS or PDS
provider or equivalent body in Scotland, Wales and Northern Ireland

(d)   a qualifying body as set out in the NHS (Primary Care Act)
1997.

IT'S NO LONGER JUST ABOUT THE DOCS

Practices will be permitted to include in their partnership, if they wish, other
healthcare professionals such as nurses, pharmacists (where there is no
conflict of interest and there is no interest held on behalf of a commercial
body), allied health professionals and non-clinical NHS staff such as practice
managers.

✓ The fundamental issue is that there must be a GP in the constitution of
the partnership and as one of the contract signatories.

Whilst it is highly desirable that every practice should have an effective
partnership agreement, the absence of such an agreement cannot prevent
the PCO awarding a practice a contract, as in the absence of an agreement
the provisions of the Partnership Act 1890 will apply.

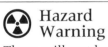 **Hazard
Warning**

There will not be a list of suitable providers along the lines of the existing
medical and supplementary lists, which are focused primarily on suit-
ability to practise. However, there will be a mechanism to prevent totally
unsuitable individuals from contracting to provide GMS, such as those
with a serious criminal history (for example, those guilty of serious
arrestable offences); those of questionable financial standing (for example, undischarged bankrupts); those with a record of serious disciplinary action by their professional body or serious internal NHS disciplinary
action (for example, a national disqualification by the FHSAA); or persons
who have been convicted of an offence in the Schedule to the Children's
and Young Person's Act 1933.

ALTERNATIVE PROVIDERS

> ✓ The PCO has maximum flexibility to commission enhanced services from other providers. The ability to commission primary medical services from alternative providers includes private sector organisations.

PCOs will be able to commission or directly provide primary medical services. This ability will sit in law alongside the GMS and PMS statutory arrangements. The changes are necessary to enable the PCO to pick up the pieces and provide services when practices bail out.

VACANCIES AND PRACTICE SPLITS

Subject to there being at least one GP in every practice, the new contract will take the form of a 'rolling' contract which will allow partners to retire and allow new partners to join the practice on the basis of continuing obligations on each of the PCO and the provider practice. It may be necessary for the contract to be linked to the practice partnership agreement in order to achieve this. In most cases this will overcome the need for a substantial variation when a provider leaves a practice or when a new provider joins a practice, subject to there being at least one GP in each partnership.

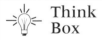
> **Think Box**
> This arrangement underlines the fact that the individual's link with 'their' family doctor is gone the same way as Dr Finlay's case book. The *practice* is now the autonomous provider of services, able to determine for itself the workforce necessary to suit the needs of its population and the desired work patterns of its workforce.

When making changes to the working practices of nurses and other healthcare professionals, the practice will be expected to involve them in the decision making and to seek advice from the relevant professional lead in the PCO.

Where there is a retirement or a new partner, the GMS provider may decide to continue to provide the services within the terms of the contract by, for example, recruiting a replacement GP or a nurse practitioner, or by increasing the hours of the practice nurse and engaging another health professional. *The flexibility is owned by the practice and the global sum will not vary unless the services are varied, e.g. if the practice opts out of a service.*

When it all goes pear-shaped in the partnership and everyone is fighting like ferrets in a sack, for example when there is a split into two groups of three practitioners each, the existing contract would come to an end and the two groups would each seek a new contract with the PCO.

Here's the nitty-gritty:

> 'There will inevitably be occasions where there is a partnership "split" resulting from a disagreement between the partners or from the expulsion of one or more partners. Whilst an expulsion in accordance with the terms of an effective partnership deed will bring about the compulsory retirement of a partner when the "rolling" principles will continue to apply, there may be a practice split which either comes about from the dissolution of a partnership at will or where various members of the partnership wish to reform into two or more separate groups. In both such cases the contract will terminate at the time of dissolution.'

Where a substantial partnership splits into two or more groups it will probably be by agreement and sufficient notice can be given to PCOs so as to permit the timely establishment of new contracts with the continuing groups. At the same time, there should be sufficient opportunity for the practice's patients to be fully informed of the new arrangements.

Where, however, there is a partnership split in a two- or three-partner practice it can often happen without any notice and considerable problems can arise in ensuring continuity of care for patients.

It is expected that in the event of partnership splits the PCO will wish to establish a temporary contract arrangement with each of the practitioners who were formerly in partnership, whilst reaching a clear understanding about patient needs and their wishes to register with one or other of the disputant doctors.

As part of the understanding, the PCO will normally agree to grant a new formal contract after a specified period of time to each of the doctors.

When a single-handed GP resigns, the PCO would still have an obligation to ensure the provision of primary medical services to that former GP's patients. The PCO could discharge that duty by entering into a contract with existing or new providers, or deliver primary medical services itself. Whilst the concept of a statutory vacancy will disappear, the LMC will be consulted about all proposals in relation to the retirement of a single-handed practitioner and greenfield sites and any existing affected patients will be kept informed.

GREENFIELD SITES

Significant increases in local population may warrant a need for additional providers of essential and additional services in an area and the PCO has an obligation to ensure provision of primary medical services to its population.

The PCO could advertise locally and/or nationally the need for a practice in the area and seek applications through a two stage process:

- first, competition between GMS and PMS practices, which would have preferred provider status
- then open competition.

The PCO would normally contract for such services through a variation to a contract with an existing GMS or PMS provider, which has a preferential right to provide such services if it so wishes. However, in stage two, the open competition stage, the PCO could commission it from another potential provider. The LMC (or its equivalent) will be consulted. To support the new arrangements around opt-outs and patient assignments, the PCO's ability to provide primary medical services itself including through PCO-led greenfield site provision would not be circumscribed by this process.

SALE OF GOODWILL

The existing arrangements prohibiting the sale of goodwill of a medical practice, including so-called deemed sales in the form of unfair partnership agreement, will continue.

CONTRACT REVIEW

The contract will be subject to a formal review process based on the principle of high trust. Although this process is distinct from the quality review process, the contract review could be carried out at the same visit so as to minimise disruption to the practice if the practice wishes. Funding for the contract review process has been built into the global sum.

The review will be based around an annual return from the practice submitted on a standard electronic pro-forma, including declaration by the practitioners/partners in the practice that they have met their statutory and other mandatory responsibilities under their contract.

> ☺ There will also be an annual review, typically involving a visit. This will include a review of the practice workload based on self-appraisal by the practice. Where a practice considers its workload so excessive that it considers opting out or closing its list, this review allows a discussion of the practice capacity. Alternatively, it also provides the opportunity for the practice to discuss with the PCO opportunities for expanding its services.

As the IT improves, so the contract management gets more interesting. The annual discussion will become strongly evidence-based, allowing the PCO to comment, offering its view of the previous year, drawing on comparable experience of workload in other practices, techniques for reducing work-load, and a discussion about what levels of support the practice might expect or desire.

> ✓ Practices will retain their option to close their list outwith this review.

At this point there will be a formal agreement if the practice wishes to withdraw from any form of service provision in line with the usual opt-out process. There will always be an opportunity for in-year discussions about contract variations, etc when required, and the review will be followed up in writing by the PCO and the practice will be given an opportunity to comment on a draft.

Either party to the contract can choose to have a representative of the LMC to support it in both the contract review and/or the quality review.

> 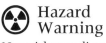 Hazard
> Warning
> Notwithstanding the PCO as the 'employer' here, the BMA says the PCOs must not neglect the informal process of developing and maintaining where appropriate a sustained empathic relationship with the practice, based on the principle of high trust and understanding of the practice's needs, pressures and aspirations, which may change in-year.

REMEDIAL NOTICES

Where the PCO believes, with reasonable cause and justification, that in any particular case the provider:

- has failed to perform the service, including failure to meet minimum standards in accordance with the provisions in the contract, or
- is otherwise in breach of the contract

. . . everyone has to start talking. The PCO and provider *will consult* or use all reasonable endeavours to agree how the breach or failure should be resolved. Either party may invite the LMC to be involved in the discussion.

> ✓ Unless the PCO believes patient safety is at serious risk or there is serious financial impropriety, the timescale will not be less than 28 days.

The PCO will issue a notice informing the practice in writing of the action to be taken, where possible, to resolve the breach or failure within a timeframe to be determined by the PCO.

Where a notice has been served and the practice does not comply within the agreed timescale, or where the breach is so serious it is not possible to resolve, there are a number of options open to the PCO.

It may:

- seek alternative provision at the cost of the original provision at the expense of the original provider until the relevant service can be re-provided by the practice within the original terms of the contract; and/or
- terminate the contract in respect of that part of the service subject to the remedial notice; and/or
- withhold and/or deduct monies which would otherwise be due and payable under the contract to the practice in respect of the element of the service not performed in accordance with the contract; and/or
- charge the practice the costs of additional administration in connection with any default on their part; and/or
- terminate the contract.

> 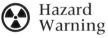 **Hazard Warning**
>
> The PCO has the right to take reasonable urgent action where patient care or safety may be at risk or where there is a serious risk to public funds.

. . . and, if the PCO has to do any of that, they will consult with the LMC.

Unsatisfactory performance by an individual GP will be dealt with either through the monitoring, appraisal and revalidation arrangements to which all GPs will be subject, or through the disqualification procedures presently set out in section 49 *et seq.* of the 1977 Act in England and Wales, sections 29 to 32E of the 1978 Act in Scotland, and Schedule 11 to the Health and Personal Social Services (NI) Order 1972.

RATIONALISING PERFORMER LISTS

This is for the bobble hat brigade and the anorak wearers . . .

At present there is provision for three separate list arrangements for GPs: the Medical List for GP principals, the Supplementary List for non-principals and locums, and the forthcoming Services List for PMS providers. Inclusion on one of these lists is a precondition of GPs performing primary medical care to patients. In England and Wales, these three lists will be merged into a single Primary Care Performers List. The Scottish Executive and the Northern Ireland Health Department will be doing their own thing – as usual.

Consideration will be given to the desirability of extending the new list over time to other primary care practitioners under GMS or PMS arrangements to reflect the practice-based approach.

RIGHT OF RETURN

PMS practices will have the ability to move to GMS on a practice basis, and vice versa.

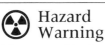 Hazard Warning
The cost of indemnity cover has been factored into the global sum and the compulsory introduction of indemnity cover will be brought in through successor arrangements to section 9 of the Health Act 1999, to reflect the practice basis of the new contract.

DISPUTE RESOLUTION AND APPEALS

When it goes bad there is 'dispute resolution' or an 'appeal'.

These two categories have different characteristics. Here they are:

> **A dispute resolution procedure** is needed to resolve issues that arise within the contract, for example a dispute as to whether a contract provision has been properly performed by either the PCO or the providers, or a dispute involving financial entitlement under the contract.

> **An appeal mechanism** is needed to deal with matters that arise outside the contract. These will largely relate to matters that deal with the relationship between the PCO and an individual GP. However, the appeal mechanism would also be appropriate where there are disagreements between the PCO and the GMS provider that do not involve matters that relate to contractual terms, obligations or rights.

DISPUTE RESOLUTION

The relevant dispute resolution procedure is dependent on the nature of the contract held by the GMS provider. The contract might be an NHS contract or an ordinary contract for services.

Contractual disputes are considered under three headings:

1   disputes where the contract is an NHS contract
2   disputes where the contract is an ordinary contract at law
3   pre-contract disputes.

These procedures will apply to all disputes that relate to contractual terms, including:

1   payments, including the global sum and quality payments, due under the contract
2   contract variations
3   opt-outs and list closures
4   contract termination
5   disputes as to contract compliance.

☺ Conciliation cannot be a mandatory precursor to formal dispute resolution. However, there is an expectation that both the PCO and the GMS provider will be encouraged to follow this route as it provides a speedier and more efficient method of resolving disputes.

As is the case with PMS, practices will have the right to elect whether or not to become an NHS body. If a dispute arises between the parties to this agreement they shall try to resolve the dispute locally in the first instance. If necessary, this should include a conciliation meeting between the provider and the chief executive of the PCO and, where it appears appropriate, could include an appropriately qualified/skilled adviser. At the time of conciliation either one or both of the parties may request the presence and assistance of the LMC.

Where the dispute is not resolved through local conciliation then the appropriate procedure will apply.

NHS CONTRACT

A practice will have the option of becoming a Health Service Body. The PCO would decide the application. If Health Service Body status were granted, the GMS contract would then have the status of an NHS contract (in Northern Ireland, a Health and Social Services contract). Such contracts are primarily governed by section 4 of the NHS and Community Care Act 1990 or equivalent and the NHS Contracts (Dispute Resolution) Regulations 1996 (SI 623/1996). It is expected that most practices would choose to enter into NHS contracts.

☺ These disputes are resolved by the Secretary of State (or equivalent) or by a person appointed by the Secretary of State (section 4(5) of the 1990 Act) or the Health Department in Northern Ireland. The FHSAA (StHA) would normally be appointed to resolve all such disputes.

Where, however, it is important to factor local knowledge into the process of adjudication, the Strategic Health Authority may be appointed. These cases involve:

• list closure
• patient assignment
• adherence to opt-out procedures.

Where the Strategic Health Authority (or its equivalent) is to be appointed as adjudicator, the Authority must, to preserve its independence, have played no part in the local dispute resolution process.

ORDINARY CONTRACTS

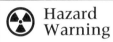 **Hazard
Warning**
Whilst the use of adjudication will be optional, its availability will be mandatory.

Where a practice opts for an ordinary contract at law they will have the option of asking the courts to resolve any resultant contractual disputes. However, it is the intention to provide an optional internal dispute resolution procedure. The process will be modelled on the existing PMS procedure, which draws heavily on the NHS contract dispute resolution procedures. Ordinary GMS contracts, which are contracts at law, will be required to include a clause that provides for dispute resolution involving binding adjudication by the Secretary of State or the Health Department in Northern Ireland. The practice therefore will have a choice of routes when there is a difference that cannot be resolved locally; either the courts or binding adjudication.

Where the dispute is referred for adjudication, the dispute would ordinarily be referred to the FHSAA (StHA). In certain circumstances, however, the Strategic Health Authority would be asked to adjudicate.

PRE-CONTRACT DISPUTES: TOLD YOU THIS GETS ESOTERIC!

In the early stages where initial contracts are being negotiated, the potential GMS provider is unlikely to be a Health Service Body. Legislation will provide regulation for the potential GMS providers to have access to adjudication in relation to a dispute that relates to the terms of a proposed GMS contract in a manner that is equivalent to the system outlined above.

The outcome of the adjudication will be binding where a contract is subsequently signed but it cannot be used to force a potential GMS provider to enter into a contract.

APPEALS

There will potentially be only a limited number of areas where a dispute might arise in an area not dealt with under the contract or pre-contract resolution procedures. These would include the right to perform GMS (i.e. matters to do with the Primary Care Performers List). Appeals will be dealt with at three different levels. In the event of an appeal against a decision made at level one, the appeal would be referred to level two.

Level one

Local resolution of those non-contractual issues. This process will allow a practice to make representations to the PCO relating to the decision that is being disputed. It is envisaged that the aggrieved practice will have access to a PCO local review panel, comprising the chairman of the PCO, an LMC or GP subcommittee-appointed member, and a lay person, but this could vary, for example according to the nature of the dispute.

Level two

Issues that are unresolved at level one. Such appeals will normally be dealt with by the FHSAA (SHA).

Level three

At the highest level appeals will lie with the FHSAA (SHA). They will deal with issues such as a practitioner's right to have his or her name entered on a Primary Care Performers List and comparable rights related to a practitioner's right to perform GMS.

LOCAL MEDICAL COMMITTEES (LMCS) AND THEIR EQUIVALENTS

Not much change, here's the detail:

> 'The role of LMCs and GP subcommittees of Area Medical Committees under the new contract arrangements will be

analogous to their existing role in each of the four countries. Under the new contract, the LMC will be involved in decisions to assign patients to practices with closed lists through the new panel arrangements. At the request of either party it could be involved in contract review or quality assessment visits, and local dispute resolution. It will also be informed of local variations to practice contracts, practice splits and the establishment of new practices including greenfield sites, breaches or failures of the practice contract, proposed commissioning arrangements for enhanced services, and re-provision of additional services when a practice has opted out.

The existing arrangements in section 44 (recognition of local representative committees) and section 45 (functions of local representative committees) of the National Health Service Act 1977 (or equivalent) will be continued in a form which will provide for the continued recognition of local representative committees and the collection from practices and the allotment to local representative committees of sums necessary for defraying the committee's administrative expenses.'

There, feel better for knowing that? I guess you do if you are part of an LMC!

PRIMARY LEGISLATION: NEW LAWS FOR OLD

An at-a-glance look at the changes in the law to enable implementation of the new contract. It is also a handy guide to some of the new responsibilities:

- repealing and completely replacing the existing GMS legislation in part II of the NHS Acts 1977 and 1978
- placing a duty on PCOs as regards the provision of primary medical services, to underwrite the Patient Services Guarantee whilst ensuring sufficient flexibility for services to develop in line with changes in medical technology and provision
- allowing PCOs directly to provide primary medical services, or commission care from alternative providers, to support the opt-out arrangements and help obviate the need for assignment of patients to closed lists
- allowing PCOs to provide support to GMS practices

- providing a legal definition of a GMS provider, and allowing them, should they wish, to be Health Service Bodies, able to enter into NHS contracts with PCOs
- setting out regulation-making powers to specify what must be included in a GMS contract, including provisions that will underpin the working definitions of essential and additional services
- providing for existing funding arrangements to be replaced by provisions comparable to those which underpin the allocation of unified budget resources, to implement the new funding arrangements, including allocation of global sum monies to practices
- rationalising the existing professional list arrangements for England and Wales.

MAKING IT HAPPEN

MAKING IT HAPPEN

All I can say is, the PCOs have got a hell of a lot of work on their plate. I'm not saying they can't do it and I'm not saying they shouldn't do it, but I am saying they need to have a very clear understanding of what they are getting into and will have to do some tough negotiating and some really thorough planning.

PCOs have a most important set of functions in relation to implementation. These range from broad strategic to detailed operational roles.

PCOs can get stuck with stuff the practices don't want to – or can't – do and they can use the contract as a lever for change.

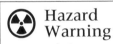 **Hazard Warning**
Some of these tasks may require skills that are not presently available in the PCO. The pressure will be on to recruit good people to do all this stuff. There will be a lot of PCOs looking for the same type of people at the same time. Recruitment will become a key issue.

The key PCO operational function is to develop and maintain effective locally held practice-based contracts. In moving away from GMS arrangements managed by the Secretary of State to a locally held practice-based contract, PCOs become the commissioners of primary care services.

PCOs will develop a range of essential, additional and enhanced services to be provided by the practice, taking into account:

- workload pressures
- the application of the opt-out rules
- the commissioning of effective alternative additional services that practices opt out of
- the commissioning of enhanced services in line with the guaranteed investment floor
- the overall level of quality that the practice expects to achieve

- the financial and other resources available to support delivery
- deployment of resources for strategic investment in premises and IM&T.

Before you relax, there is more. PCOs will also need to:

- develop an appropriate level of in-house provision of primary medical services, and
- develop a strategy for commissioning or providing out-of-hours care so that the default responsibility of GPs is removed at the earliest opportunity, and by no later than December 2004, save in exceptional circumstances and subject to agreement by the Strategic Health Authority.

 **Think
Box**

Need help?

Many PCOs may be ready for all this but many will not. Help is on the way! The Modernisation Agency is responsible for putting in place effective mechanisms to support the development of PCO competencies.

The National Primary and Care Trust (NatPaCT) Development Team, the National PMS Development Team (NPMSDT), the National Primary Care Development Team (NPDT) and the Out-of-Hours Development Team will work together with other colleagues from the Agency and with other stakeholders to develop, coordinate and establish a programme of effective support for PCOs.

Comparable arrangements will be established in the other three countries.

STRATEGIC HEALTH AUTHORITIES

StHAs have two distinct roles within the new contract:

- ensuring the effective performance of PCOs in respect of their requirements to implement the new contract, including providing developmental support and routine performance management. In particular, ensuring that PCOs are working with practices to deliver the key strategic objectives; that the guaranteed investment floor on enhanced services is delivered in each PCO; and that PCOs rapidly develop effective strategies for commissioning out-of-hours care
- discharging a limited range of technical functions as directly required of them under the new contract. These include appeals on opt-outs and

forced assignments of patients, ensuring appropriate PCO arrangements are in place for the deployment of IM&T and premises funds, and a general role in performance management.

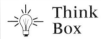 **Think Box**

Strategic Health Authorities have another little, subtle job. They will coordinate their performance management roles with those of external inspectorates such as the Commission for Healthcare Audit and Inspection (CHAI), which will be charged with assessing PCO performance and, in some countries, developing star ratings systems.

WHO DOES WHAT AND BY WHEN?

Substantial implementation will occur in **2003/04**:

	Ready for it	Got it in hand	Planning for it	Thinking about it	Help!
1 Primary and secondary legislation will be put in place, subject to Parliamentary agreement					
2 Model contracts and guidance will be prepared and published					
3 National programmes for local support will be established					
4 PCOs will review the capacity and competence they require to implement the contract and Strategic Health Authorities (or their equivalents) will performance-manage this process					
5 PCOs will prepare locally held contracts and letters in accordance with fixed UK requirements and will discuss and agree these with practices, which will also want to review their partnership arrangements in the light of new GPC guidance					
6 PCOs will develop strategies for out-of-hours commissioning and encourage transfer of responsibility to accredited providers					

Continued

	Ready for it	Got it in hand	Planning for it	Thinking about it	Help!
7 PCOs will discuss workload issues with practices, and practices will indicate which additional services they may wish to opt out of or the additional or enhanced services they may wish to provide					
8 PCOs will commission enhanced services and Strategic Health Authorities will performance-manage this spend					
9 PCOs will submit returns in a national template on transitional protection					
10 The Health Departments will allocate resources to PCOs					
11 Centralised systems will be developed to support PCOs in allocating resources to practices					
12 Revised payments for seniority payments will be introduced					
13 The definition of pensionable earnings will be changed and locum pay will be pensionable retrospectively from 1 April 2002					
14 Practices will prepare for the quality framework and be allocated preparation payments based on the Carr-Hill formula					
15 Practices supported by PCOs will take advantage of the practice management competency framework					
16 The baseline assessment of premises spend will be carried out and future spend agreed					
17 IM&T modernisation will begin, with transitional arrangements agreed nationally and discussed locally					
18 The new monitoring arrangements will be established					
19 The DDRB will be asked to set salary ranges for PCO and practice employed GPs.					

In 2004/05:

	Ready for it	Got it in hand	Planning for it	Thinking about it	Help!
20 All GMS practices will transfer to the new practice-based contract in April 2004					
21 The global sum, recalculated quarterly, and quality aspiration payments will be paid monthly. Transitional protection will also be paid					
22 It will be possible for opt-outs from additional services to occur from April 2004. Opt-outs from out-of-hours will occur, usually on a PCO-wide basis, from April 2004. PCOs will have taken on responsibility for commissioning out-of-hours by December 2004 and Strategic Health Authorities will performance-manage this process from April 2004. PCOs will be given the ability to develop direct provision of primary medical care, and to commission additional and enhanced services from alternative providers					
23 The new rules concerning patient assignments will be introduced					
24 The new performer list for England and Wales and appeals procedures will be established.					

WHEN ALL IS SAID AND DONE: THIS IS WHAT HAS TO BE DONE

Here is a list of the CONTRACTUAL and STATUTORY REQUIREMENTS that all practices have to comply with.

1 The practice provides a leaflet which is available to patients and includes:
- practice opening hours
- whether an appointments system is operated by the practice for doctor and nurse appointments

- how to access a doctor or nurse
- a description of the services provided by all members of the team and how patients can obtain them
- how to obtain repeat prescriptions
- how to make a complaint or comment on the provision of services
- a description of patients' rights and responsibilities
- how the practice uses personal health information.

2   The practice has an agreed procedure for handling patients' complaints which complies with the NHS complaints procedure and is advertised to the patients.

3   Where patients are requesting to join the practice list, the practice does not discriminate on the grounds of:
- race, gender, social class, age, religion, sexual orientation or appearance
- disability or medical condition.

4   The practice adheres to the requirements of the Medicines Act for the storage, prescribing, dispensing, recording and disposal of drugs including controlled drugs.

5   Batch numbers are recorded for all vaccines administered.

6   The practice has a policy for consent to the treatment of children that conforms to the current Children's Act or equivalent legislation.

7   The premises, equipment and arrangements for infection control and decontamination meet the minimum national standards.

8   The practice ensures that all healthcare professionals who are employed by the practice are currently registered with the relevant professional body on the appropriate part(s) of its Register(s) and that any employed general practitioner is a member of a recognised medical defence organisation and registered on a primary care performers list (or equivalent).

9   All professionals working in the practice are covered by appropriate indemnity insurance.

10 All doctors have an annual appraisal.

11 The practice has a system to allow patients access to their records on request in accordance with current legislation.

12 There is a designated individual (data controller) responsible for confidentiality.

13 If the records are computerised there are mechanisms to ensure that the data are transferred when patients leave the practice.

14 If the team uses a computer, it is registered under, and conforms to the provisions of, the Data Protection Act.

15 The practice has a written procedure for the electronic transmission of patient data which is in line with national policy.

16 The practice complies with current legislation on employment rights and discrimination.

17 All staff have written terms and conditions of employment conforming to or exceeding the statutory minimum.

18 The practice meets the statutory requirements of the Health & Safety at

Work Act and complies with the current Approved Code of Practice in Management of Health and Safety at Work Regulations.

19 Vaccines are stored in accordance with manufacturers' instructions.

20 Individual healthcare professionals should be able to demonstrate that they comply with the national child protection guidance, and should provide at least one critical event analysis regarding concerns about a child's welfare if appropriate.

21 All practices have in place systems of clinical governance which enable quality assurance of its services and promote quality improvement and enhanced patient safety. The underpinning structures within the practice will assure embedding of clinical governance through a nominated clinical governance lead.

22 For minor surgery, patients' consent to any surgical procedures including wart cautery and joint injections is recorded.

23 For vaccination and immunisation, consent to immunisation, or contra-indications if they exist, are recorded in the records.

24 For vaccination and immunisation, fridges in which vaccines are stored have a maximum thermometer and daily readings take place on working days.

25 For vaccination and immunisation, staff involved in administering vaccines are trained in the recognition of anaphylaxis and are able to administer appropriate first-line treatment when it occurs.

☢ Hazard Warning

Done all that? How do you know? Seriously, what have you got in place to audit these 25 little jobbies and prove to me, when I come and visit the practice next Tuesday, or the nice people from the PCO make a call, that it is all in place and up-to-date?

It's important, they are legal requirements. Don't do this lot, get caught and you are in deep doo-doo. These issues should be part of the practice risk management regime.

Risk management? Well there is a great book on the topic, published by Radcliffe Medical Press, written by Dr Paul Lambden and . . . – modesty prevents me from mentioning the name of his co-author! Nevertheless, the monitoring of standards is an ongoing job, like painting the Forth Road Bridge. Risk management . . . oh yes, it's the management guru version of Murphy's Law: If it can go wrong, it will!

The problem with most risk management audit is you might miss something. No excuses here – it's a nice list. Say thank you!

IN BLACK AND WHITE

The following is a copy of a letter, an exchange between the two principal players at the conclusion of their negotiations. I include it by way of balance and as evidence of what the negotiators set out to do and what they thought they had achieved.

I am grateful to them for placing it in the public domain.

John Chisholm
Chairman
General Practitioners Committee
BMA House
Tavistock Square
LONDON

26 February 2003

Dear John

New GMS Contract

I am delighted to write to you setting out the details of the new GMS contract following the outcome of our negotiations over the past 16 months. As in April 2002, I will summarise the agreements we have reached in this covering letter. Details of the new GMS contract are set out in the document *Investing in General Practice – The New General Medical Services Contract*.

The proposed new contract represents a landmark in the development of UK general practice. It provides demonstrable benefits to GMS GPs, to primary healthcare professionals, to the NHS and most importantly to patients. These, coupled with the largest sustained investment in primary care the NHS has ever made, will create the platform for a step change in improved health and health services, boosting morale and creating greater and fairer rewards for GPs.

The new contract agreement will be accompanied by investment across the UK of over £8.0bn over the coming three years. This means an average uplift in investment of 11 per cent per year, each year for the next three years. In investment terms, this deal allows for faster and more substantial proportionate growth in the primary care sector than any other area of the NHS. Within this, GPs will have the boost of significant new money for practice infrastructure (IM&T, premises and workforce); money to improve their working lives (out-of-hours arrangements, career development, appraisal, education and training, pensions etc); improved remuneration commensurate with their professional roles and responsibilities; and contribution to a reformed NHS. They will also be able to take advantage of significant additional earnings opportunities if they contribute to the expansion of the primary care sector, by developing the range of services available to patients in the community.

In summary, we have agreed:

- details of all the key aspects of the contract including pricing that builds on the framework agreement and its acceptance by the profession
- movement to a *practice-based contract* with investment for infrastructure and running costs upfront via a global sum, distributed fairly in line with the weighted needs of the patients to reflect GP and practice workload and complexity
- a system, through the *quality and outcomes framework*, for rewarding GPs and their staff for the volume and quality of the work done. This framework is designed on a strong evidence base, to reward improvements in clinical and organisational standards, and patient experience, whilst operating within a high trust monitoring system confirming GPs' professional autonomy to determine how to organise their work to achieve these standards. This framework will recognise and reward the GP's commitment to personal care, continuity of care as evidenced by good chronic disease management, and greater responsiveness to acute single episodes of care through maintenance of progress on greater choice and speed of access
- a platform for allowing *management of workload* within individual practices (through the shift of responsibility for out-of-hours care, the introduction of a changed system for managing patient allocations, the development of options to allow practices to withdraw from 'additional' service provision, typically, at times of workload pressure, the development of GP career planning, allowing GPs to take sabbaticals from practice in order to develop new skills or to replenish their energy and commitment, the promotion of multi-disciplinary working at practice level, and through a range of demand management initiatives and proposals). This contract ensures that new work is accompanied by new resources. Beyond 2005/06, this will be backed up through a process of workload review
- a strategy to *expand and develop the primary care sector* in order to allow practices to have the needs of their patients met within community and

primary settings rather than hospital, as a consequence of expanded and direct access to more specialised advice and knowledge. This will also enable those practices with ambitions to develop their range of practice-based services to provide 'enhanced' services from within the protected resource stream in the recent budget allocations

- a major *overhaul and modernisation of the infrastructure and management processes* involved in the provision of general practice (greater investment in IM&T, premises that are fit-for-purpose, greater equity of employment conditions with the rest of the NHS family, support for the development of better practice management, investment in family-friendly workforce policies, improvements to the existing pension scheme and a major drive to reduce further the bureaucracy involved in management and financial flows within general practice)
- a *programme of financial support* to help manage the transition from the old to the new contract and a sensible iteration of change, in line with the legislative timetable in the four countries, which will help practices and PCOs safely understand, prepare for and exploit the new arrangements, starting in April 2003.

This substantial package of investment and improvement in primary care, with significant earnings opportunities for GPs, provides an answer to those GPs who made it clear in your original survey that primary care could not go on without significant additional investment and that a complete overhaul of the existing contract was necessary to boost the morale of GPs, and address the problems of recruiting a new workforce and retaining the existing one.

This package is designed to support practices from all parts of the existing spectrum – whether inner city or rural and remote, single-handed or large group, well staffed or currently understaffed. This is because the new contract is fairer in the allocation of resources, allows for workload variation and management, recognises and rewards quality and outcomes, not inputs, and puts professional self-esteem and autonomy at the heart of delivery.

As to its benefits to the wider primary care workforce, this contract recognises and reinforces the multidisciplinary nature of primary care. It creates opportunities for nurses, allied health professionals, pharmacists and managers to gain from the practice-based contract, much of which will require them to be central to its delivery. It will create better corporate and clinical governance models in primary care to ensure good human resource policies are followed through in practices and will establish incentives for greater investment in basic training and continuing professional development for key practice members.

For the patient, the benefits of the contract are equally clear. The patient experience of primary care will be assessed and will contribute to the income the practice receives, creating incentives for improvements in customer care and the development of expert patient schemes. Patients will be guaranteed to receive the range of services they currently get, but with expanded choice in some service areas, improved quality and outcomes and speed of access. In terms of choice of GP and services, patients will be able to access GPs as they currently do, but will receive better information from practices about services and service changes. In some cases, patients may be able to have a choice of practice in the case of some 'additional' and 'enhanced' services. For most patients, the major benefit should come in the anticipated improvements in primary care quality they receive and the greater investment in the IM&T and physical infrastructure within the practices they are registered with.

This will, over time, reduce the need for hospital-based care for the diagnosis and treatment of most chronic disease.

There are also clear benefits in the deal for the wider NHS. The size, scale and scope of the investment in primary care, coupled with the incentives for practices to improve the quality and outcomes in treating acute and chronic health problems, now enable a shift in the focus of resources and care to primary and community settings. GPs and their staff will have greater freedom to concentrate on the delivery of high quality primary care, enabling progress to be made on tackling health inequalities and reducing unnecessary secondary care demand by keeping more people fit and healthy. Good demand management and an expansion of the primary care workforce will allow practices more time to measure and maintain the health of their practice population. The new resource formula will enable a much fairer and equitable distribution of the resources for the primary care sector and the new mechanics of its allocation will keep the money in the local practice even if GP and other staff numbers reduce. This vision of primary care is supported by many GPs who have become frustrated by the old contract and see its replacement as vital to create new incentives and rewards for GPs.

Finally, for PCOs, the new contract enables them to have a better contractual relationship with their constituent practices. One that recognises the autonomy of the practices to deliver as they best see fit but also allows PCOs to provide support to them and to organise the structures around them to maximum effect (such as workload support, out-of-hours services, protected training and development time, strategic investment in premises and effective IM&T systems).

The deal we have agreed represents a major achievement for the NHS

Confederation and the British Medical Association. Many of the things that a positive vote for this new contract would herald have been talked about but not been possible to deliver for a number of years now. I believe that GPs now have an opportunity to vote for a major programme of investment and improvement in primary care delivered through a modern, fair and principled contract. I am grateful to you and your team for all the hard work and effort that have gone into these negotiations and hope that GPs recognise the unprecedented scale of investment and commensurate earnings opportunities that will now flow.

Yours sincerely

Mike Farrar
Chair
NHS Confederation negotiating team

JUST ONE MORE?

Will it make a difference? Just one more doctor?

You see, the problem is simple – the NHS has too many customers. Great problem if you run a chip-shop. Demand-led businesses are difficult to manage but the increase in demand produces an increase in income, as the extra customers stump-up for their packet of chips.

Not so in the NHS – it is demand-led but resource-limited. The customers don't pay as they get their chips, or should I say, hips!

A big slice of the resource problem is staffing. Something like 23% of nurses are over the age of 50 and in the not-too-distant future they will be looking forward to a well-earned retirement. Big problem, especially as so much of modern healthcare is dependent on nurses doing more of what the doctors used to do. Quite who is going to do what the nurses used to do is a bit of a mystery!

Being a GP is not as popular as it once was. The new contract is aimed at making the GPs better paid (quite a lot better paid actually, estimates say the uplift in income is from £65k to around £85k), and making their working lives a bit easier. So, all these docs getting paid more for doing less means we will have to find some more docs.

Will this contract produce any more docs?

Here are some random facts from a Department of Health vacancy survey, published in November 2002. A total of 2630 GP vacancies were reported between March 2001 and February 2002, and from that total 1000 vacancies were analysed:

- 322 out of 1000 remained unfilled by February 2002
- 102 out of 1000 were vacant for more than a year
- 57% of GPs said it was more difficult to recruit now than a year ago
- 35 practices out of 550 felt they had 'compromised on experience or training' to get a partner in post
- 191 GPs retired between March 2001 and February 2002.

You can't say it makes comfortable reading. Will the contract make a difference?

According to the GP Recruitment, Retention and Vacancy Survey for England 2002, there were eight applications for each vacancy in 1999, and in 2002 it had dropped to four. Poor inner-city practices struggled the most. Three-quarters of practices said they had trouble recruiting.

And it gets worse – a large number of Asia-trained GPs, who came to the UK in the 1960s, are reaching retirement age.

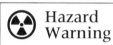 **Hazard Warning**

In November 2002, the press reported the plight of a husband and wife GP partnership in Derbyshire, who had such trouble recruiting a locum that they were forced to take separate holidays!

Let's think about this.

Will this contract bring about the dramatic changes in general practice that are needed? Will it make working in 'down-town Britain' any more attractive? If it doesn't, the people who need good primary care services the most will be most at risk.

The modifications to the pension arrangements might make some GPs remain in work for a few more years – but doesn't that just push the problem further away?

If not, what are the options? The answer might be managed services run by PCOs using a mixed economy of providers, including the private sector, technicians, paramedics and nurses.

What do you think?

Epilogue

What do you think?

Good for patients? Good for doctors? Good for the taxpayer?

I started this book cross! Now I'm sad. I am sad for primary care.

I'm a great fan of primary care. I like the idea that an independent GP, who is 'my' GP, will look out for my interests and take on the battalions of healthcare bureaucracy if I need him, or her, to.

Someone to fight my corner. A gatekeeper to stop stupid things happening and a friend in the business when the inevitable bit of foolishness creeps in. Someone who is part of the system, but a step away from the system and who can raise concerns and shout for me.

Now I fear much of primary care will be 'delivered and managed', not 'on hand as a service'.

Perhaps I have been wearing rose-tinted glasses. Perhaps I have to wake up and realise the world has moved on. Funny, really, since I like to think I have been at the leading edge of change and reform of the NHS since the mid-seventies.

I realise being a doc does not carry the status it once did. I understand there is competition in the workplace and a lot of jobs, more commodious than nursing and doctoring. I know family practice is probably unsustainable. I guess I am in a state of shock that it has come to this, at the hands of the GPs themselves. We seem to have surrendered so much, so quickly.

The docs have a new start with a new BMA Chairman, it is a watershed for them and there are huge opportunities for practice managers and PCO staff.

I hope the big brains of the NHS know what they're doing.

What do you think? E-mail me and tell me: roylilley@compuserve.com. Good luck!

☺ As we went to press, the very helpful BMA website posted two additional documents which form part of the contract agreement. No anorak's bookcase will be complete without them. Rush off and get excited at:

www.bma.org.uk/ap.nsf/Content/mpigletter

www.bma.org.uk/ap.nsf/Content/jtletter300503+

STOP PRESS

If you've already read this book you will know I make some dire warnings about the rising costs and likely difficulties for PCOs trying to manage out-of-hours care. Just as this book was going to press, this piece appeared in *The Times*, on 6 August. It seems we might be in trouble sooner than I thought!

FAMILY doctors are being offered up to £100 an hour to cover for colleagues during Bank Holidays, weekends and nights.

'Out-of-hours services, which provide cover when GPs are not working, are finding it so hard to do so that in some cases they have increased the rates of pay they offer by 40 per cent in a year.

Some doctors predict that the cost will rise further next year when GPs are able to opt out of providing out-of-hours cover, and that the cost will have to be met by Primary Care Trusts, which regulate local health services.

Latest figures reveal that doctors in Surrey are being offered pro-rata rates of £140,000 a year, an increase of 40 per cent on last year's rates of pay. Another out-of-hours service in Cleveland said that it was offering one GP £120,000 a year, and another in Harrow had increased its rates by £6,000.

The Surrey out-of-hours co-operative Thamesdoc told the medical magazine *Pulse* that it was increasing its rates by 40 per cent. It now pays £100 an hour on Bank Holidays, £65 an hour at weekends and £50 an hour for shifts during the week. The West London cooperative Harmoni said that it was increasing its rates by £6,000 to £110,000 a year.

"We will all have to take into account the going rate to get GPs to work out-of-hours," David Lloyd, external relations director for Harmoni and a GP in Harrow, said.

From December next year GPs will not have to work out-of-hours unless they wish to, and the responsibility for providing cover will pass to the trusts. Some doctors fear that this will increase the costs of out-of-hours cover yet further as more doctors opt out of the system and the trust has to pick up the bill.

GPs gained the right to opt out in negotiations this year with the Government over contracts. Much out-of-hours cover is provided at present by co-operatives of GPs, who combine to cover a number of practices. Anecdotal evidence suggests that some GPs are planning to opt out of normal hours altogether because they can now make more as a locum without the responsibility of running their own surgeries.

Richard Evans, a GP in Woking, Surrey, who works three shifts a week for Thamesdoc, said that he would not give up on his regular practice but that the pay increase would help him to retire at the age of 60.

"If there is a choice I will choose weekend sessions now as they pay more," he told *Pulse*. "It is a lot more than I get as a GP."

Tony Welch, a GP also working in Surrey, said: "The big worry is that when trusts take over the cost of providing out-of-hours cover they will not have the money to pay for it. It appears you have to pay ever more money to attract people."

The British Medical Association said that the increases were largely owing to supply and demand. "I would say the old GP contract was responsible for undervaluing out-of-hours work," Hamish Meldrum, of the BMA's GP committee, said. "What we are seeing are market forces."

"While GPs may be earning £100 on Bank Holidays, I would say the normal going rate for weekends is more like £45 an hour. While that may seem a lot, it is similar to calling out other professions during anti-social hours."

A spokesman for East Elmbridge trust said that it was concerned about the prospect of increasing wage demands. "We do not want to see the prices rocket," she said. "We are already subsidising out-of-hours quite heavily." '